SIMPLY

GOOD FOR YOU

100 quick and easy recipes,
bursting with goodness

Amelia Freer

Nutritional therapist and
number one bestselling author

Photography by Susan Bell

Michael Joseph *an imprint of* Penguin Books

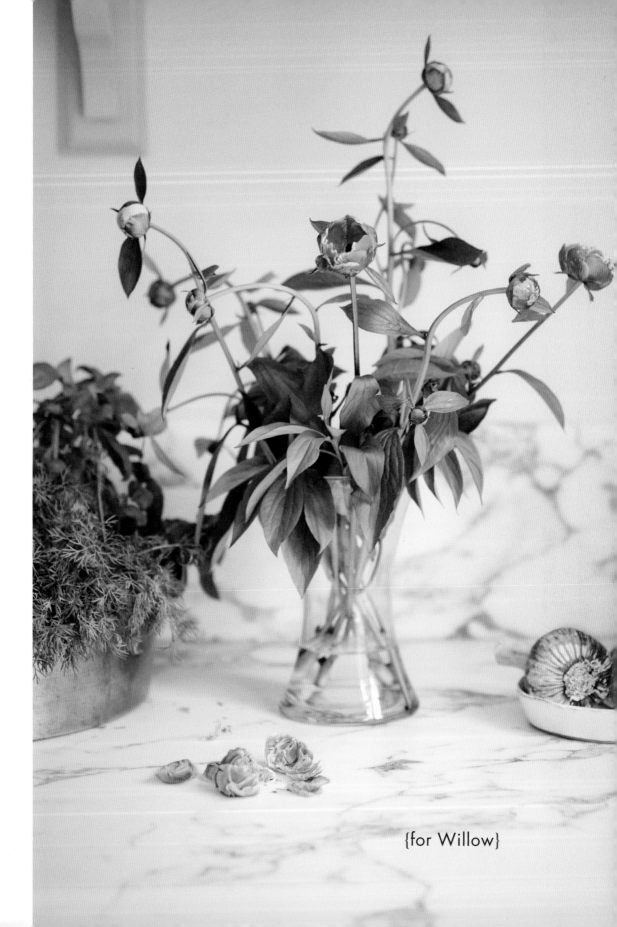

{for Willow}

contents

introduction

I am going to keep this simple. Because I think that simplicity is important in today's busy world. And if, like me, you are feeling a little weary of all the discordant advice that surrounds healthy eating, you can be forgiven for thinking that good nutrition has become too complex and faddy, and best avoided altogether. I assure you that it isn't – and it doesn't need to be. It can, in fact, be simple.

Far from being a bible of hard and fast rules, I hope that this book will instead be a refreshing dose of common sense. A real-life reference guide of varied and tempting recipes that have speed, ease, affordability and balanced nourishment at their core, while celebrating everything that is wonderful about food. After all, food is one of the greatest simple pleasures in life.

I wholeheartedly feel that healthy eating should not be equated with joyless or restricted eating (with the sensible exceptions of those who have a medical reason to steer clear of specific foods). Instead, I encourage the concept of Positive Nutrition – essentially, a focus on including plenty of the healthy foods in our diets, rather than removing the not-so-healthy. It's a mindset shift from deprivation to nourishment that is fundamental to a sustainable way of eating well, for life.

Food is more than just fuel. It is equally important to develop a balanced and relaxed relationship with food for the benefit of our social and emotional health as it is for our physical wellbeing. Being able to make food choices without experiencing guilt and to be able to relish in the pleasures of a bowl of pasta, a slice of cake, some wine, ice cream or the occasional blow-out celebratory meal are all wonderful. *And* we also need to have

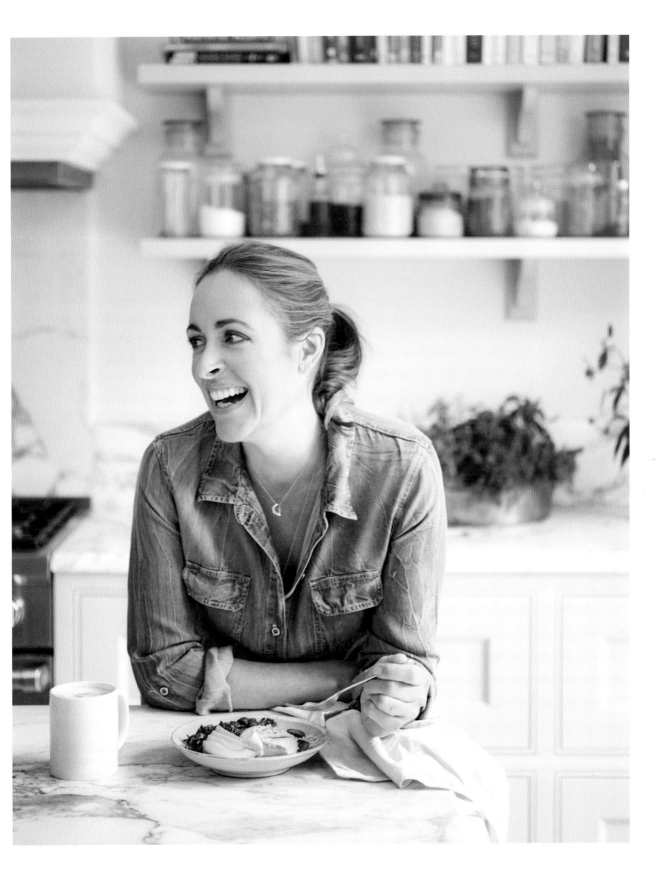

Introduction

lots of colourful vegetables, fruits, wholegrains, healthy fats and high-quality proteins too. These all equate to a balanced diet.

While the fundamental principles of a healthy diet are common among almost all of us, there is no one specific 'good diet' that is right for everyone. Just like our fingerprints, we are all unique, with diverse genetics, microbiomes, environments, cultural influences and preferences. We are extraordinary! What works for one person will be wrong for the next. There are no quick fixes either – good health and wellbeing require time and energy investment.

So, rather than following each and every diet that passes by (however persuasively marketed it may be), start to reflect what a happy, healthy mind and body means to you, and consider which small adjustments you could make from there. Keeping a symptom diary can be really helpful if you aren't in tune with your body or are finding the signals confusing. It is much easier to adopt and sustain simple changes. While planning these gradual changes, be careful not to lose sight of the bigger picture by getting too caught up in the details along the way; drinking a turmeric shot every morning won't absolve you of a fortnight's boozing, nor are vitamin supplements a substitute for real food. If you need further clarity, consider working alongside a nutrition professional to help guide you. Details on how to find a practitioner can be found on my website, www.ameliafreer.com.

Being healthy isn't just about what we eat. Eating apples and broccoli cannot plaster over years of stress, loneliness or a sedentary life. Health, pretty much like everything in life, thrives best when in balance. But I do think that the kitchen is one of the most powerful places to start to make changes to our health. A well-nourished body is able to provide the energy and impetus to make other changes, so we can start to create a positive cycle. I find the act of cooking and sharing food has, over time, become a way for me to be creative, relax and spend time with the people I love. It fuels my mind now as much as my body.

{It's a mindset shift from deprivation to nourishment that is fundamental to a sustainable way of eating well, for life.}

Of course, this isn't the case all of the time and I am aware that it isn't for most people, so I wanted this book to be really realistic in terms of how much time and energy we all have available to 'spend' on our nutrition. I am under no illusions as to how many other stresses and strains exist in day-to-day life. There inevitably will be unexpected obstacles that challenge the best of intentions, so investing a lot of time in the kitchen may not be possible. However, adopting a few simple steps, from stocking cupboards with essentials to learning a couple of go-to weeknight recipes, can pay its energy investment back many times over.

The need for speed and ease in my own kitchen has become particularly pronounced since becoming a mother. I quickly fell back into old habits as I tried to navigate the throes of early motherhood, and I am as guilty as the next person of failing to focus on self-care at times. In spite of my profession, I suffered from a bout of feeling uninspired by food. Cooking up healthy feasts were swiftly replaced with quick fixes, like a piece of toast (and full disclosure, quite a lot of Twirl bars too!). And there is nothing wrong with that occasionally, of course. It's real life. But I had a niggling feeling that I could nourish myself a little better (and consequentially *feel* better for doing so) tapping away at my consciousness.

So I chose to start simply, as I have advised my clients for years. For me, it started with toast. I made a promise to myself that no matter how tired I was, or even if I was making it with a single hand (usually with a sleeping or crying baby in the other), I'd throw a couple of extra ingredients on top to make it a complete meal. And by complete, I mean it contained some sort of vegetables, protein (such as an egg) and healthy fat (a drizzle of olive oil or some seeds). That's all. Simple. And it grew from there. I named them my 'hero toppings' and started adding them to anything and everything – from baked potatoes and rice cakes to flatbreads and pasta. You'll find my hero toppings on page 108.

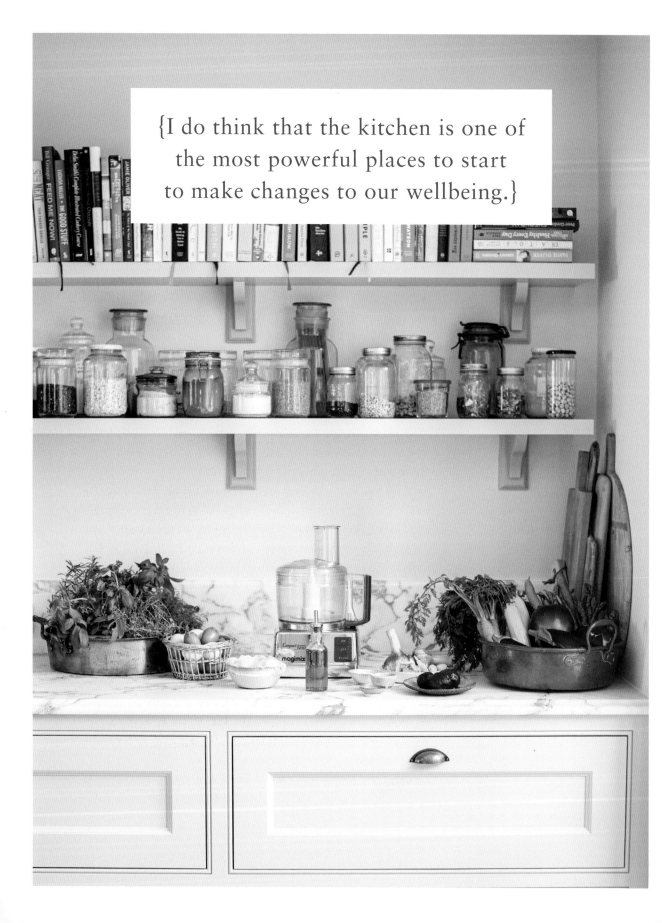

{I do think that the kitchen is one of the most powerful places to start to make changes to our wellbeing.}

I also felt motivated to ensure that the time I invested in the kitchen preparing food for my young daughter could feed us all, well, as a family. The notion of cooking separate baby food just didn't make sense to me as this meant she ate well but I just grazed on leftovers (which is something I have heard so many of my clients struggle with, so I knew I wasn't alone). Food was shared from the start and we reaped the benefit in time, cost and nutrition. This book holds the recipes for the majority of the meals that we have been eating, as a family, over the past couple of years. They are unashamedly simple because that is reflective of real life, and how most of us eat every day.

Bringing all of those common experiences together, I have focused here on what we know is beneficial for us to eat, translated into quick and simple dishes to fit into real life, and I'm giving you the freedom and scope to adapt each recipe to suit your own needs. Be creative and playful – time spent in the kitchen can be reframed to be relaxation time rather than another chore. I know cooking from scratch might not always be possible, but taking a few simple steps towards a healthier diet will make a huge difference over time. Just one more portion of vegetables a day provides our body with an additional 3,650 portions over ten years. Now that's food for thought!

There are very few recipes here (perhaps apart from a couple of the baking ones) that cannot lose an ingredient or accept a substitution here or there. You are encouraged to be inventive, swapping in ingredients that you favour, or have to hand, especially seasonal alternatives. You'll also find plenty of variety in the dishes, including meat, fish, vegetarian and vegan options, so I hope there's something for everyone. Above all don't sweat the detail. Everything in this book is quite simply, good for you.

healthy eating on a budget

With an ever-increasing strain on our household finances, finding ways to eat well without it costing a small fortune is a top priority for many. Thankfully, with some canny planning and a little ingenuity, it is absolutely possible to create delicious, healthy meals on a limited budget.

1. Avoid ready-prepared ingredients

If budget, rather than time, is your main priority, avoid buying a lot of prepared ingredients. Instead, wash, peel and chop fruit and vegetables, soak and cook dried pulses and grains (you can do this in bulk and freeze them, cooked, in batches*), season meat yourself, prepare sauces and dressings from scratch, and avoid buying too many ready-meals.

Making packed lunches and snacks to take with you and always carrying a refillable water bottle are also huge cost savers.

2. Embrace frozen produce

Frozen produce is often cheaper, and no less nutritious, than buying fresh. Plus, there is less risk of food wastage. Some supermarkets hold a much broader range than others, though, so you may need to shop around. Take a look at Kitchen Staples & Shortcuts on page 26 for a list of favourites.

*
The exception to this is red kidney beans, which I would always recommend you buy ready-cooked, as they can be toxic if not prepared properly.

3. Minimize food waste

Meal planning and sticking to a set shopping list can help prevent waste, but it's useful to have a few strategies up your sleeve for using up 'sad' ingredients too:

VEGETABLE SOUP: Great for any odds and ends of cooked or raw vegetables you have lying around. Sauté an onion and a little garlic, add the chopped veg, pour over just enough stock or bouillon to cover, and simmer until tender. Blend and you're done. Also see my 'Bottom of the Fridge' Vegetable Stew on page 214.

FRITTATA: The sheer variety of ingredients that can be thrown into a frittata makes this a staple meal. Bits of cheese, grated or chopped veg or herbs, leftover pulses or chopped meat – anything goes.

STIR-FRIES: Good for using up vegetables, chicken or prawns.

GRAIN SALADS: Leftover cooked grains (with the exception of rice, which I don't keep because of the potential risk of food poisoning), can be transformed the following day with a handful of chopped greens/herbs, tomatoes, cucumber, lemon juice and a glug of olive oil.

OVER-RIPE FRUIT: Can be stewed into a compote (delicious with a dollop of yoghurt and nuts or seeds for breakfast), or frozen for smoothies.

4. Know your shops & markets

Find out about local market dates and times (traders often sell off produce cheaply towards the end of the day), supermarket bargains (and their potential discounting times) and independent shops with great offers.

I go to Middle Eastern and Arabic shops or the 'world food aisle' of bigger supermarkets for cheap bulk spices, dates, nuts and tahini, for example. Online retailers may also offer good discounts on bulk food cupboard staples.

A few supermarkets and online companies are now offering 'wonky' vegetable boxes, which are a more cost-effective alternative to their cosmetically perfect equivalents.

Getting shopping delivered, or signing up for a weekly vegetable box, helps avoid going to the shops and thus being seduced by the displays and offers of 'nice, but not essential' things – which can really add up.

5. Buy in season

I know this is far from an original piece of advice, but the price difference between seasonal and out-of-season foods, particularly fruit and vegetables, is enormous. There are plenty of resources online to help you know when different produce is at its peak.

6. Grow your own, if you can

If there is any chance that you could grow some of your own food, this can potentially make a sizeable impact on your outgoings on fresh fruit and vegetables in the longer term, whether it's just a few herbs on a windowsill, or going so far as to apply for an allotment. Cut-and-come-again salads seem to give me the best return on investment!

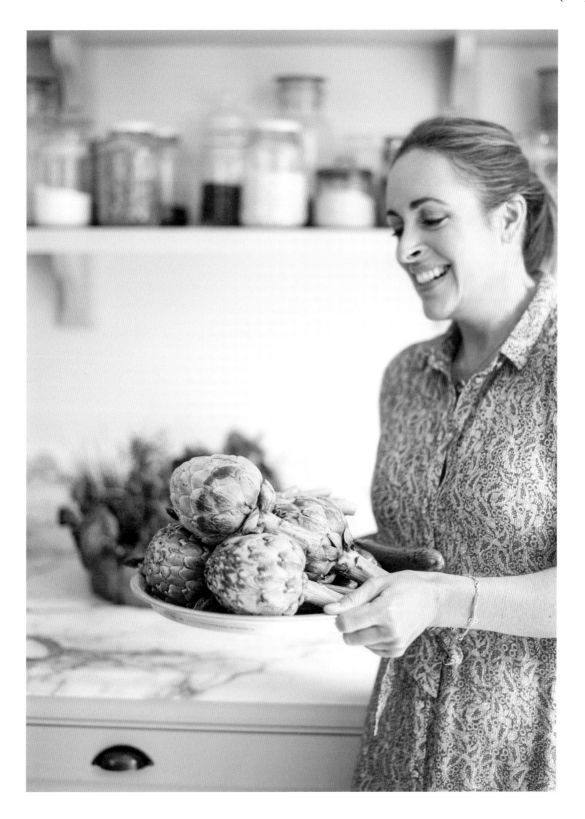

Healthy eating on a budget

{14}

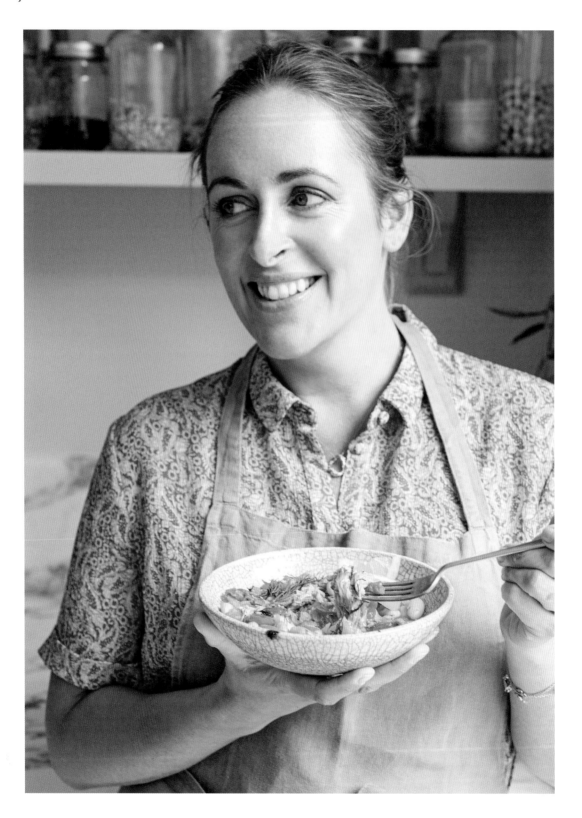

Healthy eating on a budget

7. Vary protein sources

A big dent in the weekly food budget can come from buying enough good-quality protein sources, especially fish and meat.

- You can spend less on meat per portion by choosing the cheaper cuts. The best person to speak to about this is your local butcher, if you're lucky enough to have one, although here are a few pointers on various economical cuts to look out for:

FOR ROASTING (Beef) Brisket, rump, (Lamb) Shoulder, (Pork) Belly, neck.

FOR STEWING (Beef) Shin, chuck or blade, leg, (Lamb), Shoulder, scrag and middle neck,(Pork) Chump, cheek.

FOR STEAK (Beef) Flank, rump, (Lamb) Chump, (Pork) Chump

- Choose more plant-based proteins (such as nuts, seeds and legumes), free-range eggs or natural yoghurt. Buying less meat overall is not only potentially good for the environment, but can also save money.

- If you've got a freezer with space to spare, consider speaking to local farmers or farm shops about buying your meat in bulk. Many will sell a box of cuts at a discount, such as half a lamb, and you'll know exactly how that animal was raised and where it came from.

- Bulk out meat dishes with additional pulses or vegetables. Lentils, finely chopped mushrooms and grated carrots work particularly well in mince dishes, for example, and a big stew can be bulked up with the addition of plenty of chopped vegetables, beans and the odd potato.

ingredient
swaps

There are very few recipes in this book that require the exact ingredients (or even the exact amounts) specified. Many will happily take substitutions, according to what's in season, what you have to hand, or what you prefer. The only exception to this is baking, where culinary chemistry tends to require a little more precision.

Here are a few ideas for ingredient swaps that I often use, both in the upcoming recipes and in my cooking in general.

APPLE CIDER VINEGAR   Any vinegar can pretty much be substituted with another, but I tend to reach mainly for white wine vinegar, balsamic vinegar or lemon juice if I'm out of 'ACV' (and vice versa).

BREAD   Choose any bread you like. I tend to go for a minimally processed gluten-free option, but fermented sourdough, wholegrain, spelt and rye are also great choices.

DRIED FRUIT   You can substitute dates in recipes with the equivalent weight of dried figs, raisins, sultanas or dried apricots. Be aware that they do all have quite separate and distinct tastes, and figs will also change the texture, as they have seeds. It might offer an interesting variation on the theme, however.

FISH   The key with fish substitutes is matching fillets approximately by size/thickness (and therefore cooking time) and also by type. If in doubt, ask your fishmonger.

- **White fish fillets:** hake, haddock, cod, pollack, monkfish, whiting, ling

- **Oily fish fillets:** wild salmon, mackerel fillets, trout fillets, sea trout, sardines

- **Small, round fish:** whole mackerel, small trout, sea bass, sea bream

- **Small, flat fish (usually fillets):** lemon sole, plaice, Dover sole

- **Smoked fish:** smoked salmon, smoked mackerel, smoked trout

FLOUR

Flours can often be tricky to substitute because they each have specific properties. If you are OK with gluten, you can substitute any of the gluten-free flours for their equivalent standard flours I suggest (i.e. plain, self-raising, bread). I sometimes use buckwheat or gram flour instead of plain flour for savoury recipes, and buckwheat flour makes great pancakes. I also use ground almonds and polenta, which are particularly good for baking.

If you don't have any self-raising flour, you can make it yourself by sifting together 1 teaspoon of baking powder per 120g plain flour.

FRESH CHILLI

Depending on how hot the fresh chillies are – I tend to work with ½ teaspoon dried chilli to each small fresh one. Obviously you can adjust this to your personal preference. And leave them out if serving to small children (although Willow likes chilli).

FRESH GINGER

Substitute ¼ teaspoon of ground ginger for every 1 tablespoon of grated fresh ginger. Peeled fresh ginger stores very well in the freezer, and is easy to grate from frozen with a good grater.

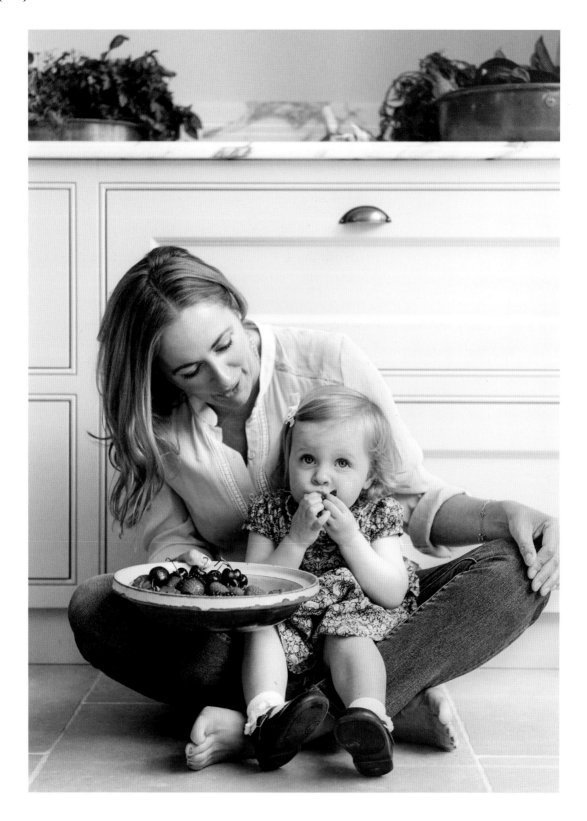

Ingredient swaps

FRESH HERBS Most fresh herbs can be swapped around, according to what's available. It will change the taste of the dish, but some-times that results in an improvement. However, I would typically stick within the following categories to avoid overpowering a dish inadvertently.

- **Soft herbs:** parsley, coriander, rocket, basil, mint

- **Woody herbs:** rosemary, thyme, bay, sage

You can substitute 1 tablespoon of the chopped fresh herb for ½ teaspoon of the dried herb.

FRUIT Many fruits can be substituted for each other in the recipes, and it is often worth experimenting to see what works for you. However, to maximize your chances of success, I would generally stick to swaps within certain categories (as they tend to share flavour profiles, water content and/or textures).

- **Berries:** strawberries, blueberries, raspberries, blackberries

- **Citrus:** lemon and lime (very interchangeable, including in savoury recipes), grapefruit, orange, clementine, mandarin

- **Hard fruit:** apples, pears

- **Stone fruit:** cherries, plums, damsons, nectarines, peaches, fresh apricots

- **Exotic fruit:** mango, papaya, pineapple, banana

MILK You can generally use any milk of your choice in recipes – dairy (cow's, sheep's or goat's) or dairy alternative (such as almond, oat, or coconut). It is best to use unsweetened. If you avoid dairy, look out for plant-based milks that are fortified with calcium. I try not to use ones that contain added emulsifiers.

NUTS AND SEEDS

These are pretty much interchangeable. For example, you can use sunflower seeds instead of pumpkin seeds. Hazelnuts, pistachios, cashews, chopped Brazils or walnuts instead of almonds, etc. There are lots of possibilities, according to what you have available to you and your personal preferences. The only exception here is chia seeds, which struggle to be substituted as they are often used specifically as a thickener. Chia seeds can be purchased cost-effectively, in bulk, online.

OILS

I try to keep things as simple as possible when it comes to fats and oils in the kitchen, as it is a bit of a minefield and there's been a lot of confusion in recent years. I mainly cook with light olive oil, or sometimes coconut oil (especially good for curries), and then keep an organic, extra virgin olive oil or rapeseed oil for drizzling and dressing. If you're OK with dairy, then organic butter and ghee is lovely from time-to-time. I generally avoid 'vegetable' oils or sunflower oils, margarines and other processed fats (especially anything containing trans fats).

ONIONS

I use onions and garlic all the time as the 'base' of my savoury cooking. You can buy handy bags of ready-chopped onions for the freezer (a great cheat for the busy cook), but if you've neither fresh nor frozen onions, you can use leeks, spring onions or shallots as an alternative.

PASTA AND NOODLES

I tend to use a mixture of different pasta types, especially when cooking for my daughter. If you're OK with gluten, then whole-wheat or spelt pasta is a good choice. If you're gluten free, look for buckwheat, brown rice, pea or red lentil pasta. Cooking times vary, so follow the instructions on the packets.

POTATOES

Any other starchy vegetable can usually stand in for a potato; sweet potato, parsnip, carrot, beetroot or squash, for example. You might just need to adjust the cooking times.

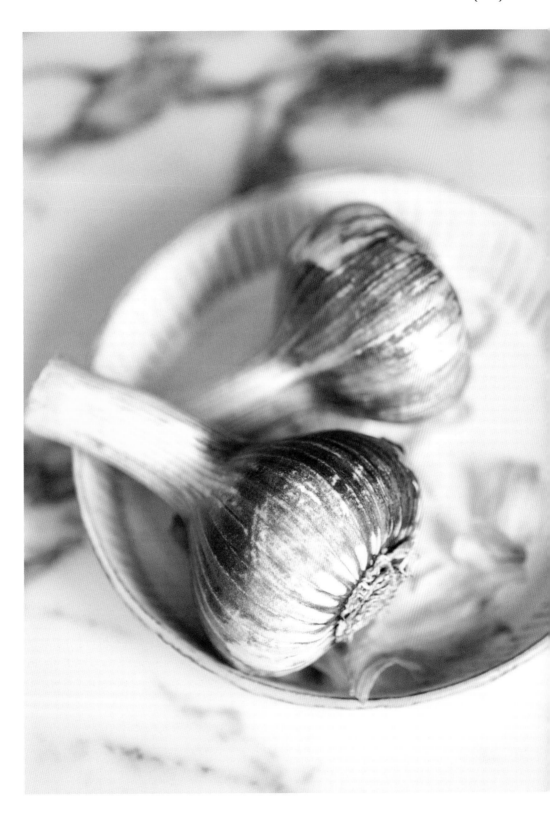

Ingredient swaps

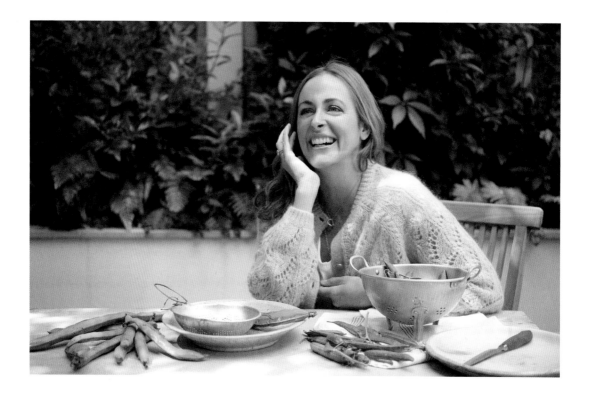

PULSES AND LEGUMES   Many of these can be swapped with each other. Tins of butter beans/chickpeas/kidney beans/cannellini beans, etc. in place of each another. You could also use broad beans or peas instead of tinned pulses (thawed first if frozen).

SALAD GREENS   Some recipes will specify watercress or rocket or spinach, these can absolutely be swapped with any salad leaves of your choice, or indeed fresh green herbs (such as parsley, basil and coriander), according to your personal preference. I generally recommend the darker greens over plain lettuce, where possible, for maximum nutrients.

SPICES   I tend to substitute within the following groups:

- **Sweet:** cinnamon, ginger, mixed spice, nutmeg

- **Spicy:** chilli powder, cayenne, hot paprika, curry powder, pepper, smoked paprika

- **Fragrant:** cumin, ground coriander, garam masala, curry powder

- **Colourful:** turmeric, saffron, paprika

STOCK   Stock can be swapped (chicken/beef/fish/vegetable) with the equivalent volume of another. Instead of slow-cooked bone stock, you could use a stock cube, or bouillon powder, made up according to the packet instructions. Stock is sometimes referred to as 'bone broth'. If you use a cube or powder, I suggest you reduce or avoid adding extra salt to the finished dish as they are often high in sodium already.

SWEETENERS   Most liquid sweeteners (honey, maple syrup, coconut nectar, etc.) can simply be substituted in the same quantities. Remember to avoid using honey if you're cooking for children under 1 (in which case, I use maple syrup). I generally avoid synthetic or artificial sweeteners. Otherwise, I use organic normal sugar, or dried fruit (puréed dates work well in baking, or very ripe mashed bananas), although this sometimes affects the taste or texture of the finished dish. A little experimentation in the kitchen is always a good thing.

VEGETABLES   Most vegetables can be swapped around, according to what is in season, and what you enjoy. I generally try to keep their textures fairly well matched where I can (i.e. broccoli or cauliflower, aubergines or courgettes, carrots or beetroot, spinach/greens/chard/kale), but apart from that, I use what I have, not what the recipe instructs.

YOGHURT   I often use plain coconut yoghurt, but you can also use Greek/natural cow's, sheep's or goat's milk yoghurt too (or a good organic soy).

Natural, unsweetened, full fat cow's milk yoghurt is the best choice if you're OK with dairy, as it contains a good amount of protein (helping to balance blood sugars and keep you feeling full for longer) as well as probiotic bacteria (good for gut health). If you struggle digesting cow's milk yoghurt, you could try goat's/sheep's milk yoghurt instead, or organic vegan options such as soy, coconut, cashew or almond – all of which are available in large supermarkets (however, they are a more expensive option). Avoid yoghurts with added flavours or sugars, and choose the ones with the fewest ingredients.

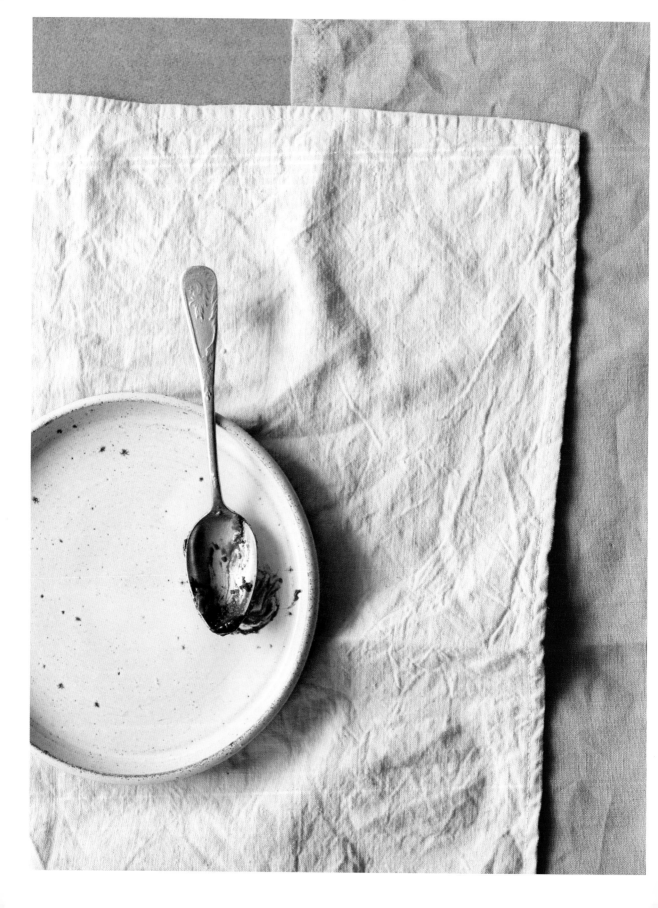

kitchen kit

The following kitchen utensils are the things that I use day-in, day-out, and really make it quicker and easier to cook from scratch on a regular basis. Some things are definitely an investment (or a practical gift guide), but are worth it in the long run.

- A heavy chopping board and sharp knives (a small preparing knife, chef's knife and bread knife are my most used)*

- Microplane grater (for zesting citrus, grating ginger and garlic)

- Lemon juicer

- Vegetable peeler

- Garlic press

- Measuring jug or cups

- Set of light mixing bowls

- Fish slice, flexible rubber spatula, whisk and wooden spoons*

- Sieve and colander*

- Large frying pan, with lid*

- Three sizes of heavy-bottomed saucepans, with lids

- Large casserole dish, with lid*

- 2-layered steamer saucepan*

- Large roasting tray (which can double up as a baking tray)

- Ceramic or enamel oven dishes: small and medium

- Loaf tin (helpful if you're baking bread regularly)

- Slow cooker or Instant Pot

- Food processor

- Stick blender (with an electric whisk attachment too)*

- Electric weighing scales

- High-speed blender (this is superior to a food processor for making soups, smoothies and sauces) – although you can get away with just a stick blender for most recipes

- Selection of heatproof glass storage containers, with lids

All these items are available to buy through my online shop at www.ameliafreer.com.

*These are my essentials, if you are not sure where to start building your kitchen kit from.

kitchen staples & shortcuts

These are the staples I keep in my kitchen, as well as some of the shortcuts and 'cheat' ingredients I use when time is really tight–although it's not really cheating, just practical! Since becoming a mother, I have certainly learned not to judge myself, or worry about using these shortcuts when I need to. They might be a bit more expensive, but sometimes I am happy to pay the price to make things a bit swifter. These items/brands are available to buy via my online shop, www.ameliafreer.com.

Cupboard

STAPLES

Oats, quinoa, buckwheat, pasta, bread, dried herbs and spices, bouillon powder, cocoa or cacao powder, flours, baking powder, olive oil, vinegars, salt, pepper, tinned or jarred fish (tuna, sardines, anchovies), tinned or jarred cannelini, tomatoes, passata, tinned or jarred cooked pulses such as lentils, butter beans and chickpeas, packets of milled flaxseed and various seeds.

SHORTCUTS

- Cooked beans, lentils or chickpeas in glass jars or tins (I like the ones from Brindisa).

- **Cooked lentil/quinoa pouches:** Lots of supermarkets now offer pouches of cooked lentils, quinoa and other whole grains. They last for ages in the cupboard (without needing refrigeration), and can be a very handy staple to grab when you need to boost a meal quickly. (I like the ones from Merchant Gourmet.)

- **Jarred tomato passata/chopped tomatoes:** Jars or tins of great-quality chopped tomatoes or tomato passata are definitely a staple in my cupboard.

- **Jarred cooked peppers:** Cooking and peeling peppers is a real faff. I just don't bother any more, but buy jars of ready-peeled and roasted peppers in olive oil instead. Drain and rinse them well before using, and roughly chop them into an otherwise bland salad, or blend them into a soup or a tomato and pepper sauce.

- **Garlic purée:** Peeling and crushing garlic cloves fresh does undoubtedly produce a better flavour, but it also creates an extra step of washing-up and preparation and I think these little things can often put people off. So using a good garlic purée, kept in the fridge once opened, can save valuable time and won't really have a huge impact on the final dish.

Just in case you didn't know (which I didn't until recently), you can press unpeeled garlic cloves directly through the garlic press. It takes a little extra effort, but once through, the flesh comes out of the holes while the skin is left behind in the press. Easy. Thanks to Jamie Oliver for this tip!

Freezer

STAPLES   Frozen peas, ice, lots of labelled leftovers.

SHORTCUTS

- **Frozen berries/fruit:** I don't buy fresh berries when they are out of season, as they are often very expensive, and can rack up air miles and time from field-to-fork (potentially reducing their nutritional value). Instead, I freeze my summer harvest of foraged or homegrown blackberries, blueberries, strawberries and raspberries, or buy them directly from supermarkets to use in the winter months. I often buy exotic fruit (mango, pineapple, papaya, etc.) frozen too – it's cheaper and less likely to go off.

- **Frozen beans of all varieties:** While we may all have a stash of frozen peas in our freezer most of the time, can I also suggest that you pick up bags of green beans, baby broad beans and soy beans when you see them? They all freeze well, and are much less effort to cook than preparing from fresh.

- **Frozen avocado:** I was a little sceptical about this when I first came across it, but frozen avocado is great if you use it to make smoothies, sauces or to add to soups. It is cheap, easy to throw into a dish and avoids that 'unripe, unripe, unripe, overripe' pattern that we all know too well.

- **Frozen fish and shellfish:** Some types of fish do not freeze particularly well (salmon being one of them, I think), but others don't seem to suffer from the process. If you can find unsmoked, frozen mackerel fillets, for example, these cook very well straight from the freezer. Or wild, white fish fillets (such as haddock or cod), which I always cook in a sauce from frozen (or they tend to go too dry). I sometimes also buy frozen fish pie mix – it is a useful ingredient to have to hand if you find yourself cooking for friends last-minute. The same goes for frozen, sustainably caught prawns. Alternatively,

I find you can make any fish freeze more successfully by transforming the fresh fillet into a quick fishcake (see page 162), and freezing it like that instead.

- **Frozen chopped onions:** Keep a bag of frozen, chopped onions and garlic in your freezer and you're a step ahead for many of my dishes.

- **Frozen chopped herbs:** I will usually freeze a glut if I have grown them myself, but all sorts of herbs are now available in the supermarket freezers too.

Fridge

STAPLES Milk (of choice), eggs, feta, salad, vegetables, fruit, yoghurt.

SHORTCUTS

- **Washed salad:** The ease with which I can sort a meal if I have a bag of prepared salad to hand is certainly time-saving. If I am preparing my own, I will wash the whole lettuce or bag of greens at once, and spin it dry, then leave it in the salad spinner with the lid on inside the fridge.

- **Ready-prepared vegetables:** These are definitely more expensive to buy than whole vegetables and may lose some nutrition through storage, but if this is what it takes to help you cook more quickly and pack in the vegetables that your body needs, then of course go for it. The alternative to buying the vegetables ready-prepared is to make extra when you do have a moment, and just leave these in a covered box ready for more time-stretched moments. Wash everything, peel carrots, dice roasting veg, etc.

BREAKFAST

1}

Wholefood smoothies

Breakfast smoothies can be a very quick and easy way to support our overall nutrition. I put all the ingredients into my blender jug the night before and leave it in the fridge ready to whizz together in the morning. That way, I know I've nourished myself with at least one portion of vegetables, some fresh fruit and protein, without thinking too hard about it. But personally, I struggle with the taste and texture of protein powders, and so was keen to find some tasty 'wholefood' alternatives to help me stay full until lunchtime and prevent a blood-sugar roller-coaster ride. Here are four for you to try.

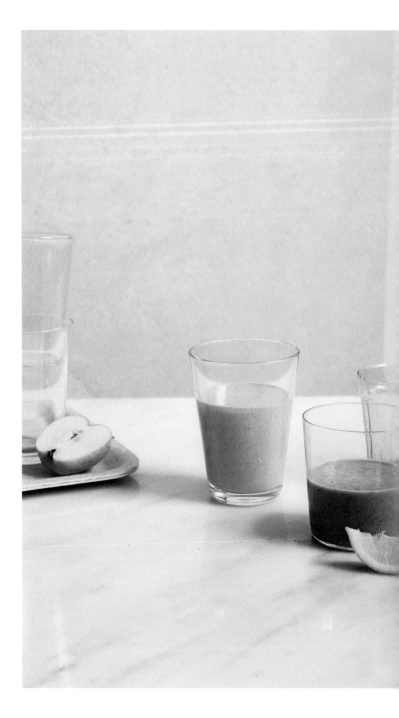

golden

{Serves 2}

150g natural goat's, sheep's or almond yoghurt (unsweetened)

150ml milk of choice

150ml water

2 bananas

2 teaspoons ground turmeric

1 teaspoon ground cinnamon

2 tablespoons almond butter

a pinch of freshly ground black pepper
(helps the turmeric to be absorbed)

Blend all the ingredients together until smooth. Drink immediately.

green

(vegan)

{Serves 2}

4 tablespoons hulled hemp seeds

a small handful of spinach,
roughly chopped

½ a cucumber, roughly chopped

10g fresh ginger, peeled and chopped

1 apple, cored and roughly chopped

180ml coconut water or plain water

a squeeze of lemon or lime juice

Blend all the ingredients together until smooth. Drink immediately.

tip: These recipes, and the smoothies on the following pages, are a great place to start, but do experiment and play around with different flavours and combinations. I have a simple formula for a nutritionally balanced smoothie:

+ 1 portion of fruit (to avoid too much sugar)
+ 1 portion of veg (baby leaf spinach is the mildest to use)
+ 1 portion of protein (nuts, seeds, nut butter, natural yoghurt or protein powder of your choice)
+ other flavours, ice and liquid to taste

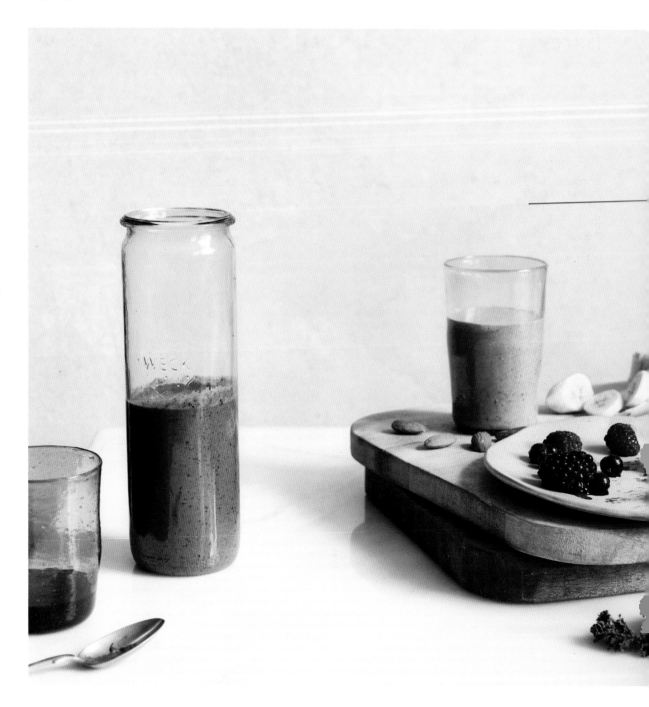

berry
(vegan)

{Serves 2}

125g frozen berries

300ml milk of choice (I use almond for this)

a small handful of chopped kale
(blanched in hot water for a minute,
then rinsed in cold water)*

4 tablespoons hulled hemp seeds

½ teaspoon vanilla extract

Blend all the ingredients together until smooth.
Drink immediately.

chocolate
(vegan)

{Serves 2}

1 medium banana

1½ tablespoons cacao powder

450ml almond, hazelnut or cashew milk

1 heaped tablespoon chia seeds
(approx. 30g)

30g almonds, soaked if possible
(soak for 30 minutes in boiling
water and drain before blending)

Blend all the ingredients together until smooth.
Drink immediately.

*
tip: Pop the kale into a sieve and pour boiling water
over it. Then run it under the cold tap. This should be
enough to soften the kale and make it a bright green.

bircher muesli

{Serves 2}

This Bircher becomes my go-to breakfast in warmer months. It takes just a minute or two to throw together before bed, and each batch will last 2 to 3 days. I have given you the ingredients in volume measurements, as I can rarely be bothered to get out my scales to make it, but the weights are there too if you prefer to use them. Use whichever milk and yoghurt you prefer. Multiply the recipe as required to make a bigger batch.

Base mixture

1 cup of rolled oats (100g)

1 cup of milk or water (250ml)

4 heaped tablespoons yoghurt

2 tablespoons chia seeds

Mix everything together well in a large bowl. Leave covered in the fridge overnight to soak.

Topping suggestions

Liven up the base mixture with any combination of the following. They can be added at the time you make the base or thrown on top in the morning. Bircher is incredibly forgiving – and you'll soon learn how you best like yours. Each combination is the recommended amount per portion.

~ 1 cup of chopped mango (approx. 150g) (I use frozen chunks – they defrost well overnight in the fridge) and a small handful of almonds.

~ 1 cup of berries (approx. 150g) (I use frozen if not in season).

~ ½ a banana, ½ teaspoon ground turmeric and 3 tablespoons pumpkin seeds.

~ 1 grated apple, ¼ teaspoon ground cinnamon and 2–3 tablespoons mixed or ground seeds (best if left to soak overnight).

~ ½ teaspoon vanilla extract and 2 tablespoons cacao nibs.

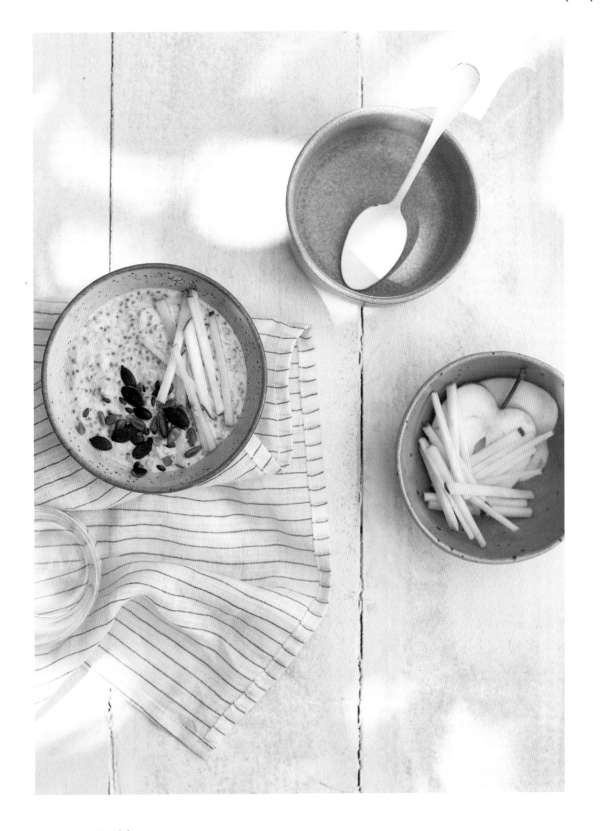

Chapter 1 ~ Breakfast

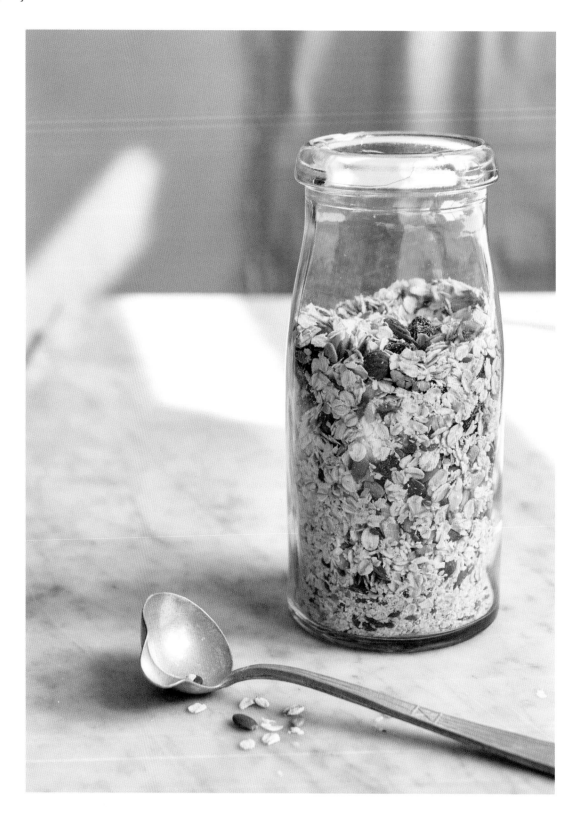

coconut
muesli
(vegan)

{Makes 15 portions}

When you need something instant for breakfast, having a jar of this muesli to hand can make life a little easier. It keeps for ages, and usually works out more economical than many 'artisan' or gluten-free muesli boxes you see for sale. It will keep for 2 months in an airtight container. Use whichever nuts and seeds you prefer.

450g whole rolled oats

300g mixed seeds (I use a shop-bought packet which contains linseeds, pumpkin seeds and sunflower seeds)

150g whole nuts or chopped nuts

150g desiccated coconut

90g raisins

Mix all the ingredients together, and transfer into an airtight container.

Serving suggestions

~ Add cold milk of choice and enjoy 'plain'.

~ Soak overnight in milk or water and top with chopped fresh fruit.

~ Mix with yoghurt and berries for a quick Bircher.

~ Add warm milk, or warm gently on the hob with water or milk for a seedy fruit porridge.

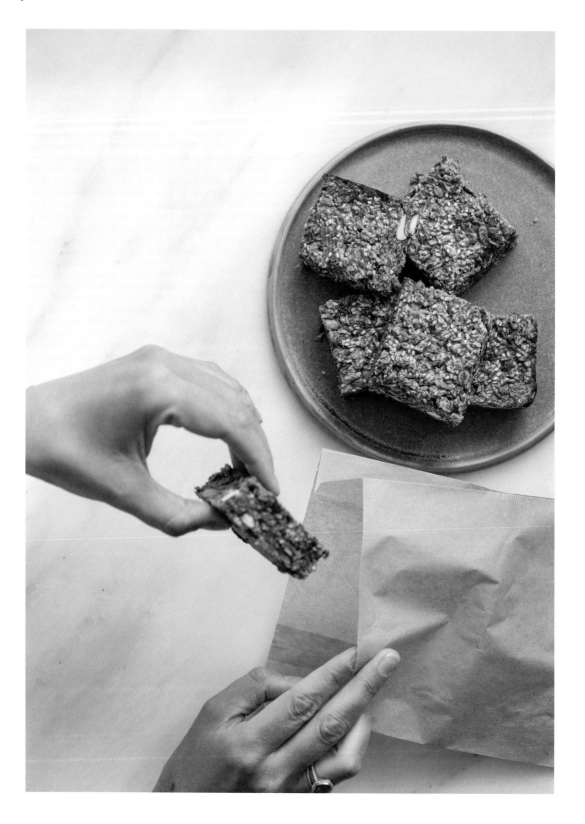

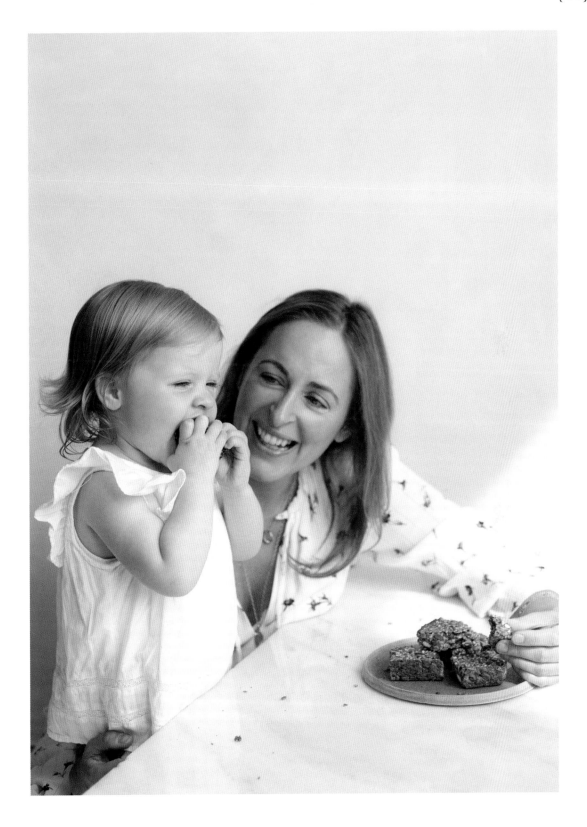

Chapter 1 ~ Breakfast

beauty bars
(vegan)

{Makes about 10 slices}

These bars are packed full of skin-boosting vitamins and minerals from all the nuts and seeds. They can be enjoyed as a grab-and-go breakfast, or as a quick snack after work or school. This recipe is pretty versatile, so you can mix the nuts and seeds to use up whatever you may have lurking in the cupboards. Will keep in an airtight container for 3 days, or longer in the fridge.

flavourless oil, for greasing
100g pitted dates
2 tablespoons chia seeds
200ml hot water
80g nut butter
150g mixed seeds
100g oats
50g almonds

Preheat the oven to 180°C/160°C fan. Grease the base and sides of an 18cm square brownie tin and line with baking parchment.

Soak the dates and chia seeds in the hot water for 10 to 15 minutes, until they get nice and plump and the liquid has cooled down.

Blend the dates and chia seeds and their soaking water with the nut butter to make a smooth paste. Mix this paste with the remaining ingredients and press into the lined tin with the back of a spoon.

Bake for 30 to 40 minutes, or until the top is golden brown and it feels firm when pressed.

Cut into slices while still warm and in its baking tin, but allow to cool completely before turning out.

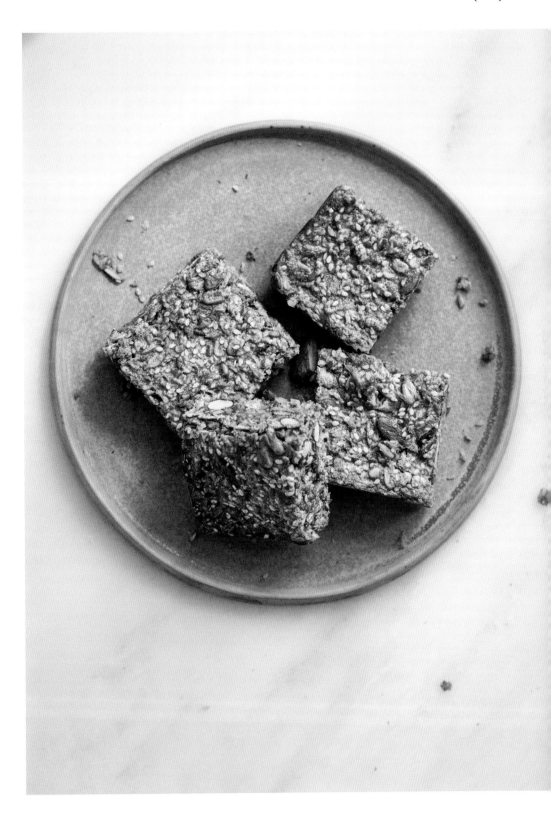

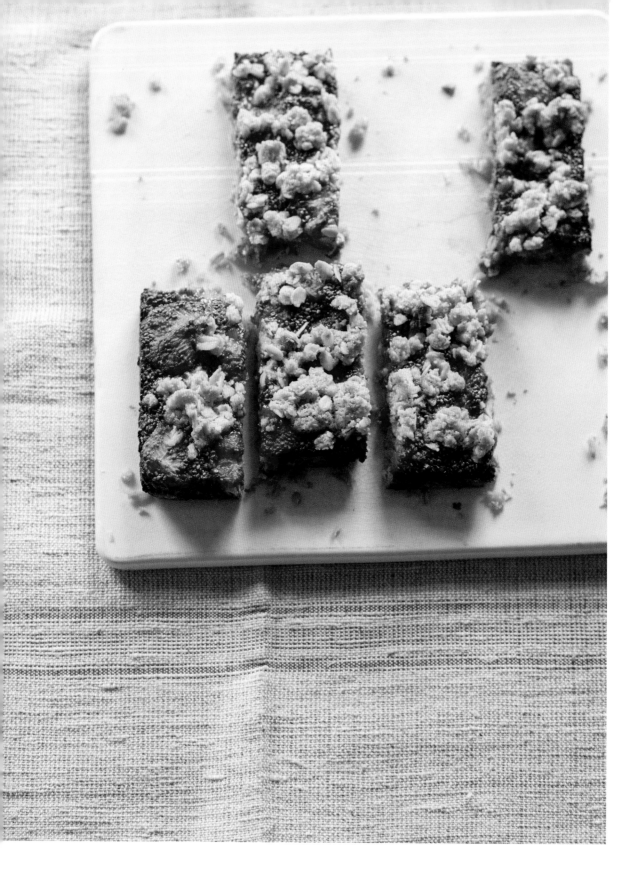

fruity breakfast crumble bars

(vegan)

These are great for grab-and-go breakfasts. They're also a winner with kids and make a good after-school snack. All berries work well for the filling.

{Makes 8 bars}

For the filling

170g frozen strawberries

1 tablespoon water

2 tablespoons chia seeds

1–2 tablespoons maple syrup (to taste)

For the base and topping

1 chia 'egg' (1 tablespoon chia seeds + 2½ tablespoons water)

90g jumbo oats

45g ground almonds

45g oat flour (just whiz oats in a blender)

75ml maple syrup

75ml coconut oil, melted

Preheat the oven to 200°C/180°C fan. Line a 15cm square cake tin with baking parchment.

To make the filling, put the berries and water into a saucepan and heat over a low heat for 8 to 10 minutes, using a wooden spoon to gently break the berries up so they are less chunky but still not smooth. Add the chia seeds and 1 tablespoon of maple syrup. Remove from the heat, taste and add more maple syrup if desired.

Make the chia 'egg': mix together the chia seeds and water and leave to sit for 5 minutes.

Place the oats, almonds, oat flour, maple syrup and coconut oil in a bowl. Mix together, then scoop out 2 tablespoons of the mixture and set aside (this will be the crumble topping).

Add the chia egg to the bowl and mix to combine. Press the mixture into the lined tin and top with the berry jam. Scatter the 2 tablespoons of mixture you set aside over the top and bake in the oven for 30 minutes.

Allow to cool completely before cutting into bars.

banana
bread
(gf)

{Makes 10 slices}

Halfway between a cake and a bread, when sliced and toasted (even from frozen), it makes a lovely breakfast, topped with a dollop of yoghurt and some squashed fresh berries. It's not too sweet, which I enjoy as I am definitely more of a savoury person in the mornings, but if you wish, you could add a tablespoon or two of maple syrup or honey to the mixture before baking.

flavourless oil, for greasing

4 very ripe bananas, peeled

3 large eggs

200g buckwheat flour

2 tablespoons olive oil

80g ground almonds

1 teaspoon mixed spice

a pinch of sea sea salt

80g chopped walnuts

2 teaspoons baking powder

Preheat the oven to 200°C/180°C fan. Grease a 900g/2lb loaf tin and line it with baking parchment.

Mash the bananas with a fork in a large bowl. Add the eggs and mix well. Add the buckwheat flour, olive oil, almonds, mixed spice, salt and walnuts, then sieve in the baking powder. Mix well.

Pour into the greased and lined loaf tin and bake for approximately 30 minutes, or until well risen, golden brown and a skewer inserted into the centre comes out clean.

tip: This recipe is great for using up any bananas that are turning brown. They make it even more sweet and moist.

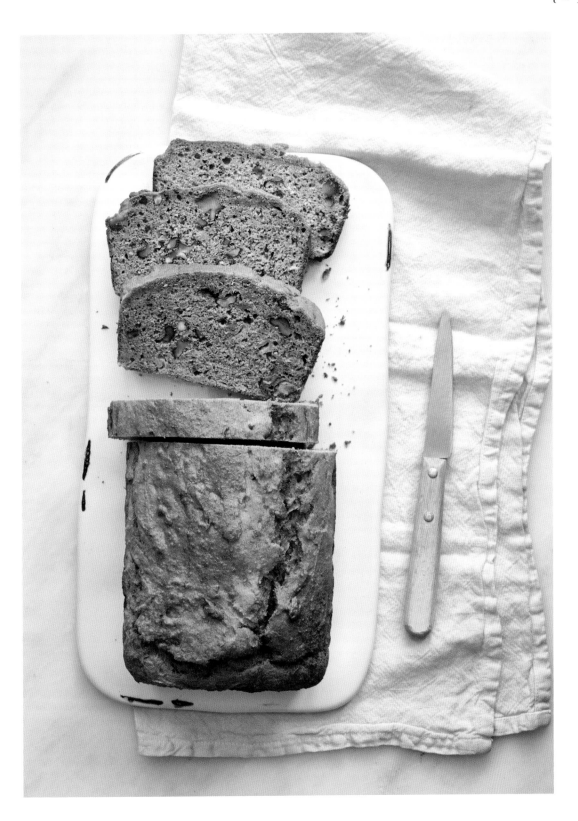

veggie bread

(gf)

{Makes 1 large loaf}

I make a variation of this bread at least once a week. It keeps for a few days and toasts brilliantly. As a soda bread, it can be baked immediately after mixing, as it doesn't need time for the yeast to rise. Other variations I have tried are grated carrots, finely sliced spinach or broccoli florets that have been pulsed in the food processor a few times. Store in the fridge for up to 3 days, or slice and freeze, then toast when you need.

375g gluten-free bread flour (I use Doves Farm brown bread flour)

4 large eggs

2 teaspoons baking powder

1½ level teaspoons sea salt

3 tablespoons olive oil, plus extra for greasing

3 medium courgettes (approx. 500g), coarsely grated

Preheat the oven to 220°C/200°C fan. Brush a 900g/2lb loaf tin with olive oil and line the base with a strip of baking parchment.

Mix all the ingredients together in a bowl until well combined. Tip into the greased loaf tin, flatten the top, and bake for 50 to 60 minutes, or until golden brown and a knife poked into the centre comes out clean. Turn out on to a rack to cool completely before slicing.

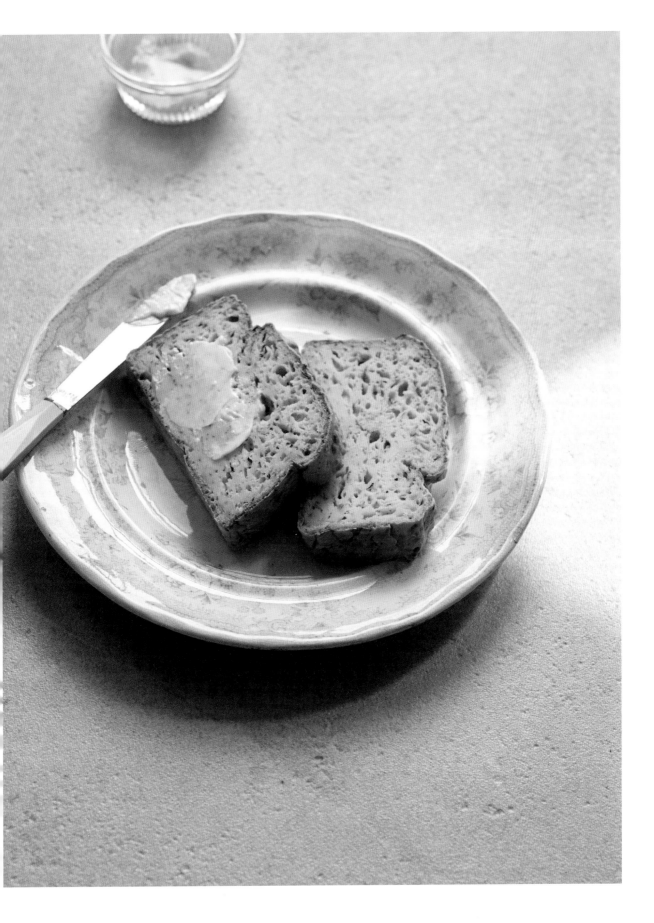

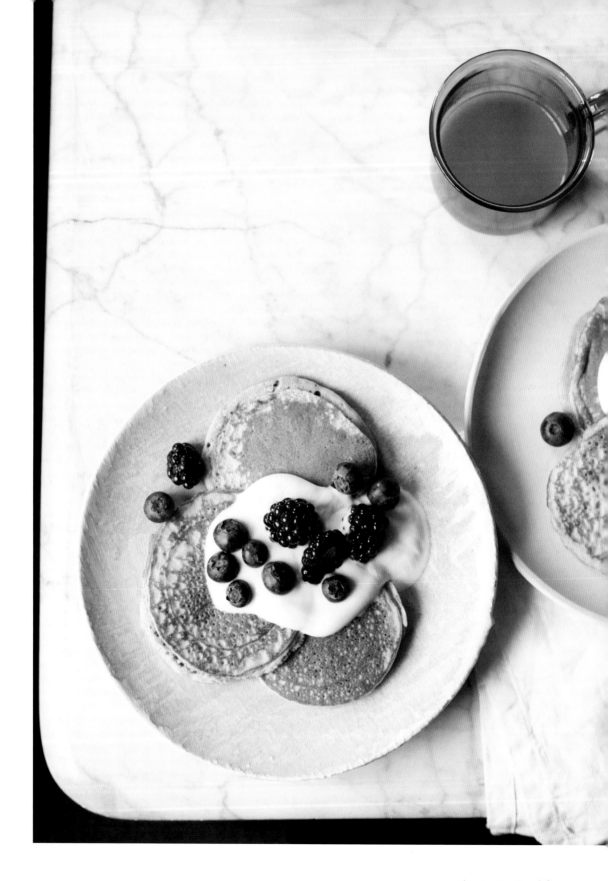

protein
pancakes
(gf)

{Serves 2}

This mixture can be whizzed up the night before and left in the fridge overnight ready for the morning. Play around with the flavours. Substitute vanilla for mixed spice or cinnamon, and serve alongside whichever fruit is in season. Chopped plums, nectarines, apples, pears or cherries would all be delicious.

1 large banana

3 medium eggs

75g ground almonds

1 teaspoon vanilla extract

To serve

a dollop of coconut yoghurt or natural yoghurt

a handful of berries

Blend the banana, eggs, almonds and vanilla together in a high-speed blender until smooth.

Preheat a non-stick frying pan over a medium heat. Fry small pancakes (roughly 8cm across/2 tablespoons of batter per pancake), flipping them over when bubbles appear around the edges. Once the other side is cooked, remove from the heat on to a serving plate.

Serve with a dollop of coconut yoghurt or natural yoghurt, and a handful of berries.

yoghurt bowls

Yoghurt, fruit and nuts make one of the simplest breakfasts. Here are four of my favourite options.

pistachio & apricot

{Serves 2}

6 dried apricots

juice and zest of 1 large orange,

340g natural, unsweetened yoghurt (or kefir)

30g pistachios, roughly chopped

Soak the dried apricots in the orange juice and zest overnight, or gently heat them together in a pan until plumped and juicy. Blend to a purée (I use a hand-held stick blender).

Swirl the apricot and orange purée through the yoghurt, and top with the pistachios.

tip: If you don't have time to soak the apricots overnight, blend them, unsoaked, with the orange juice and zest. Almonds work well if you don't have pistachios.

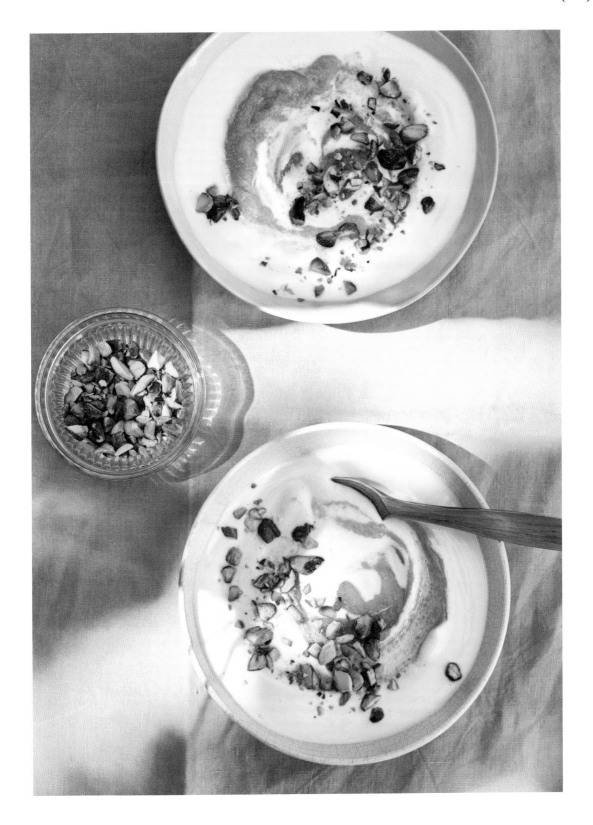

Chapter 1 ~ Breakfast

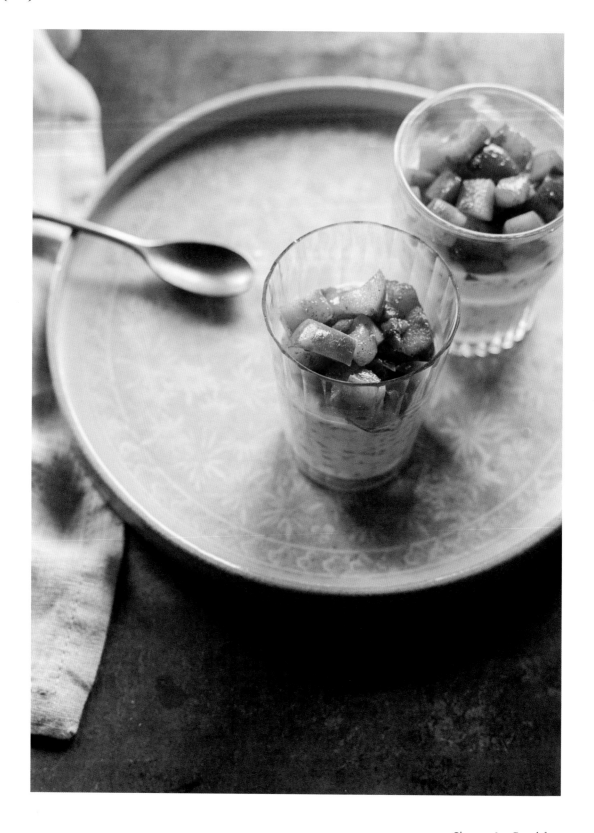

gut-friendly

{Serves 2}

Stewed apples are a great source of prebiotic fibre for your gut, while live yoghurt provides friendly probiotic bacteria. The two combined make what is called a symbiotic food. Which also happens to be delicious. Win, win!

1 large eating apple, cored and diced (skin left on)

1 large pear, cored and diced (skin left on)

½ teaspoon mixed spice

6 tablespoons mixed seeds

340g natural, unsweetened yoghurt (or kefir)

In a small saucepan, stew the apples and pears (with a dash of water to stop them sticking) with the spice. This should take around 10 minutes or so. Allow to cool.

Mix the seeds into the yoghurt (or kefir).

Spoon the yoghurt into a small bowl or glass. Top with the stewed apples and pears.

berry jam

Chia jams are very easy to make. We enjoy it spread on toast, spooned on to scones (see page 248), stirred through porridge or, on busy days, simply with yoghurt. The chopped almonds provide an extra dose of essential nutrients and healthy fats.

{Serves 2}

300g frozen berries

1 tablespoon chia seeds

1–2 teaspoons honey

340g natural, unsweetened yoghurt (or kefir)

30g almonds, roughly chopped

Defrost the berries in a small saucepan over a medium heat, adding a splash of water if necessary. Once completely defrosted, stir in the chia seeds and honey, then leave to one side to cool. The chia seeds will absorb the liquid and make the mixture thicker, like a jam.

Put the yoghurt into a bowl and spoon over the chia jam. Sprinkle the chopped almonds on top.

tip: Chia jams last in the fridge for 3 days and also freeze very well to make extra, if you like.

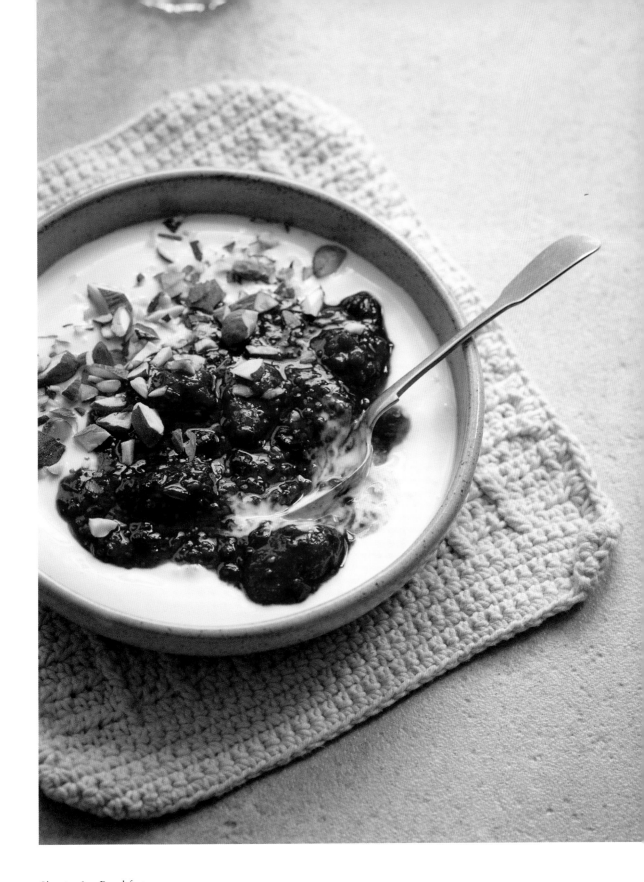

fig & hazelnut

{Serves 2}

This is a divine breakfast to enjoy in summer, when fresh figs are ripe and available. If they are really soft and sweet, you can forgo the baking first, simply tear them directly into the yoghurt. Out of season, soak dried figs overnight in a little water to plump them up.

60g hazelnuts, roughly chopped

4 ripe figs (or dried figs), diced

1 teaspoon honey/ maple syrup

½ teaspoon ground cinnamon

340g natural, unsweetened yoghurt (or kefir)

Preheat the oven to 200°C/180°C fan (I usually make this when I have the oven on anyway). Line a baking tray with baking parchment.

Combine the chopped hazelnuts, figs, honey and cinnamon together and mix until well coated. Place on the lined baking tray and bake for 10 minutes.

Divide the yoghurt between two bowls. When the fig mixture has slightly cooled, spoon it on top of the yoghurt and serve.

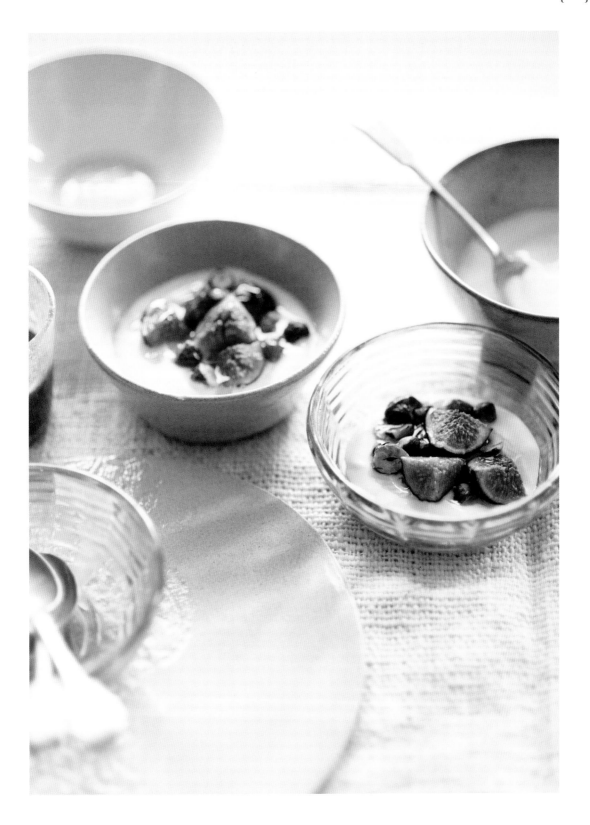

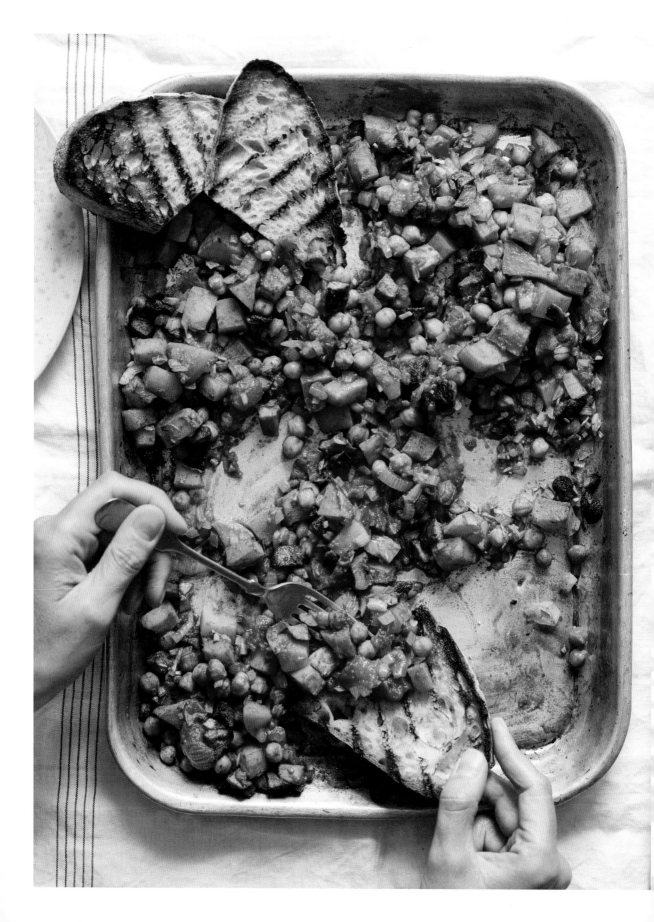

butternut baked beans

(vegan)

{Serves 4}

This recipe makes a large quantity, and it keeps well in the fridge for 2 to 3 days, so you can enjoy it for other meals. The flavour gets better and better. Very economical, and extremely versatile – it's my favourite kind of cooking. For breakfast, I enjoy this with some spinach and a poached egg, for example. It's also great cold for lunch with salad leaves and crumbled feta. Or for supper, with roasted chicken and steamed greens. If you don't wish to make such a large portion, just halve the amounts of butternut squash, onion and mushrooms.

1 butternut squash, peeled and cut into 1cm cubes

2 medium onions, peeled and diced

2 cloves of garlic, crushed

200g mushrooms, roughly diced

1 x 400g tin of chickpeas, drained and rinsed

3 tablespoons olive oil

3 teaspoons smoked paprika

1 x 400g tin of chopped tomatoes

sea salt and freshly ground black pepper

Preheat the oven to 200°C/180°C fan.

Put the squash, onions, garlic and mushrooms into a large roasting tray, along with the chickpeas. Drizzle with a little olive oil and sprinkle over the smoked paprika. Use a large spoon to mix everything well, ensuring that the vegetables and chickpeas are evenly covered with the paprika oil.

Bake for 30 minutes, stirring halfway through if you get the chance, until everything starts to soften and caramelize at the edges. Add the tinned tomatoes and stir through. Then return the tray to the oven for another 10 minutes.

Season with salt and pepper to taste before serving.

egg & vegetable traybake

{Serves 6}

This one-pan traybake is a lovely weekend option to have cooking while you are doing other things around the kitchen. It is quite forgiving if you are a few minutes delayed. It will keep in the fridge for up to 3 days, and makes for a very quick meal.

olive oil

1 red pepper, deseeded and diced

150g mushrooms, diced

1 courgette, diced

10 eggs

100ml unsweetened milk of choice (or chicken or vegetable stock)

1 teaspoon ground turmeric

1 teaspoon ground cumin

sea salt and freshly ground black pepper

1 x 400g tin of chickpeas, drained and rinsed

50g spinach, roughly chopped

Preheat the oven to 180°C/160°C fan. Oil a deep-sided baking tray or small roasting tray (30 x 20cm) well – including right around the edges.

Place the diced peppers, mushrooms and courgettes in the tray, and roast for 30 minutes, or until softened.

Whisk the eggs with the milk, turmeric and cumin, and season with pepper and salt (use around 1 level teaspoon if you are not using a stock cube, just a pinch if you are).

Mix the chickpeas and chopped spinach into the roasted vegetables (in the same tray), then pour over the whisked egg mix. Place the whole lot back in the oven for a further 20 to 30 minutes, or until the top is browned and it is set all the way through.

Cool completely, then slice into 6 pieces.

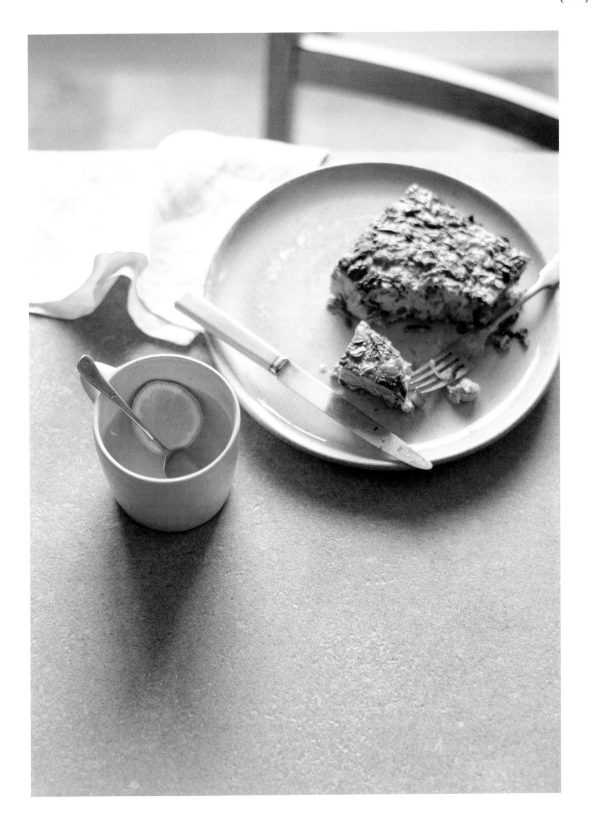

breakfast pizza

'Pizza – for breakfast!?' Yes! And it's not all that strange when you consider the ingredients: bread, tomatoes, spinach, mushrooms, egg – all well-known breakfast foods. But there is something deliciously decadent about combining them into a 'pizza' that makes it feel like a morning treat, albeit a quick and easy one. Willow and I have actually eaten this at all times of day. She loves to be involved in the decorating process!

{Serves 4}

4 Yoghurt Flatbreads (see page 109) or 4 wholemeal pitta breads

4 teaspoons fresh pesto

40g baby leaf spinach

4 cherry tomatoes, quartered

4 button mushrooms, sliced thinly

½ a red onion, peeled and thinly sliced

½ a red pepper, deseeded and sliced

olive oil

sea salt and freshly ground black pepper

4 small free-range eggs

a grating of cheese

Turn the grill on to medium high.

Spread the flatbreads or pittas with a little pesto. Put a thin layer of spinach on top and dot the cherry tomatoes, mushrooms, onions and red peppers over the top. Drizzle with a little olive oil and season with salt and pepper.

Place under the grill for 3 minutes, just to soften the vegetables. Make a well in the middle of each flatbread, then break an egg into each one. Sprinkle over the cheese, then put back under the grill for about 5 minutes, until cooked as desired (I like my yolk just a little runny).

tip: Don't worry if the egg doesn't stay in place – it still tastes good!

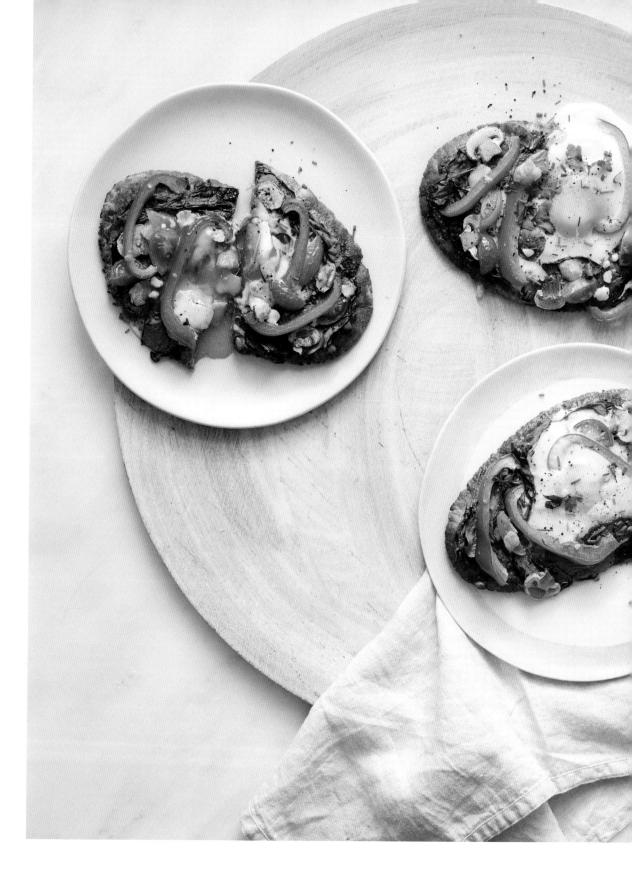

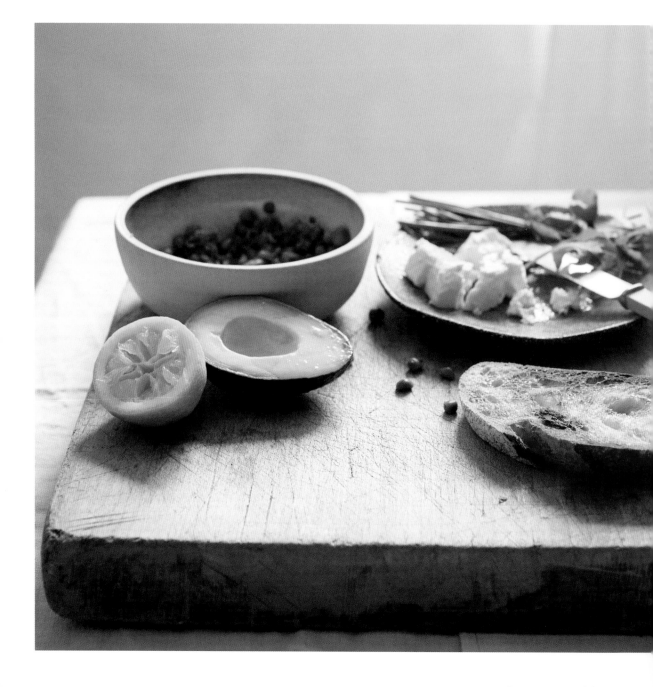

green toast

Toast is a go-to breakfast staple for many of us, but the toppings we choose can impact its nutritional value. Here, peas provide fibre and plant-based protein (and are something most of us have in the freezer), feta adds a tangy saltiness, and protein to keep us full, and avocado lends creaminess along with healthy fats. Any extra topping makes a great lunchbox option, with a handful of rocket, a few cherry tomatoes, and whoop – two meals for the time it takes to make one.

{Serves 2}

2 slices of bread of choice

4 tablespoons frozen peas

10g feta, crumbled

½ a large avocado, or 1 small avocado, peeled and roughly chopped

2 tablespoons olive oil

juice and zest of 1 lemon

a handful of rocket

a small handful of fresh chives

freshly ground black pepper

Put 2 slices of bread of choice in to toast. Put the frozen peas into a cup and cover them with boiling water. Leave for a minute, then drain.

Mash the feta, avocado, peas, olive oil and lemon juice together.

Put a little rocket on top of each toast, then spoon over the feta, avocado and pea mash.

Top with chives, and sprinkle with freshly ground black pepper and a little lemon zest.

mackerel & spinach on toast

{Serves 1}

The long-chain Omega-3 fats found in oily fish are so important for our health. Smoked mackerel is a simple way to eat more, as it is ready-prepared and lasts a good while in the fridge.

1 large or 2 small slices of toast of choice

1 fillet of smoked mackerel, skin removed, flesh mashed with a fork

juice of ½ a lemon, plus a little zest to garnish

olive oil

a handful of baby spinach leaves (approx. 40g)

freshly ground black pepper

chilli flakes (optional)

Put the bread on to toast. Mash the smoked mackerel, lemon juice and 1 teaspoon of olive oil in a bowl.

Drizzle a little olive oil over each slice of toast.

Put the baby spinach leaves into a bowl of hot water for a second to wilt, then drain, squeeze out excess water and pat dry with kitchen paper. Lay the spinach on the slices of toast (or just add the raw spinach, if you are short of time).

Top with the mackerel mash. Sprinkle with a little lemon zest and freshly ground black pepper and scatter over some chilli flakes, if you like.

This also works well stuffed into a warmed wholemeal pitta bread, to eat as a sandwich.

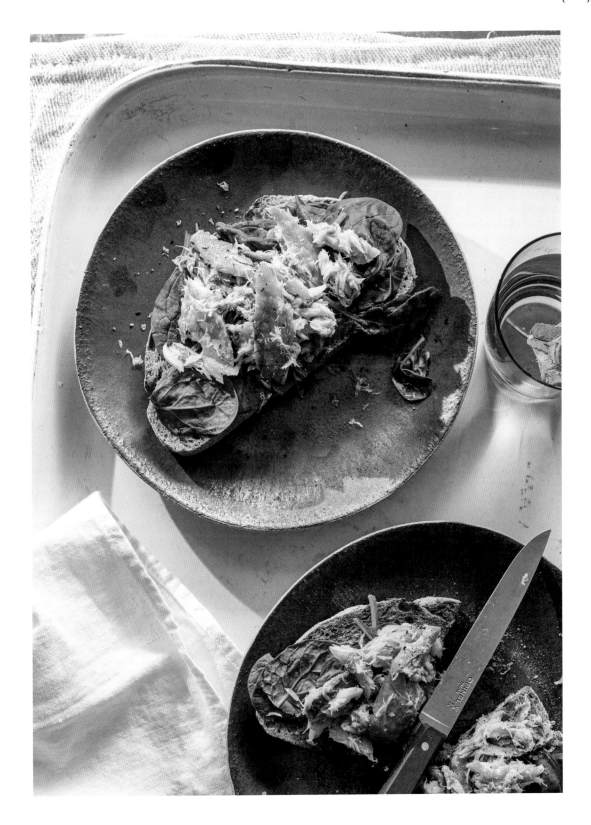

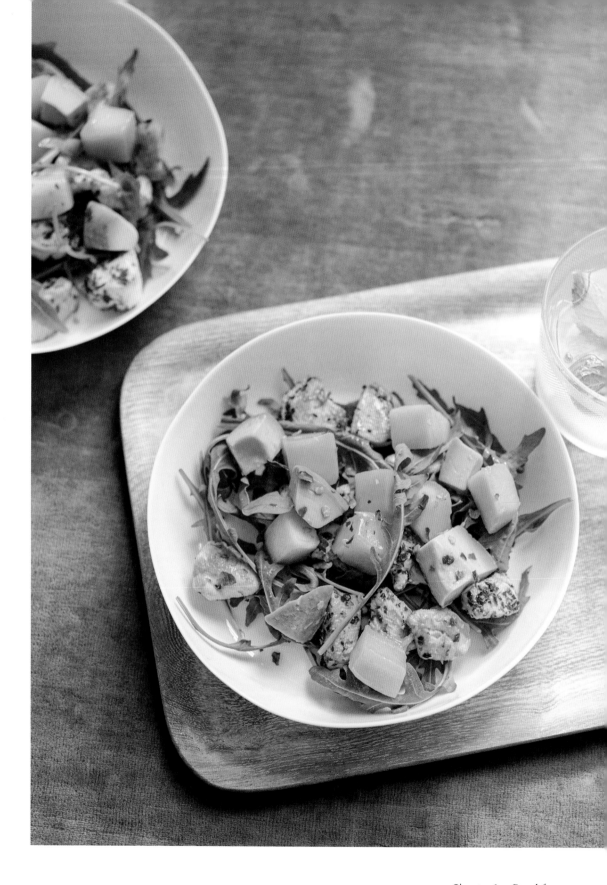

chicken & mango breakfast salad

{Serves 2}

When I first suggest to clients that they try chicken for breakfast, they are often a little bit wary. But most love it. It can of course work for any meal, but I urge you to think outside the box and try some different, more unusual things for breakfast occasionally. You too may be pleasantly surprised.

1 tablespoon olive oil or coconut oil

1 small skinless chicken breast, diced

1 teaspoon dried mixed herbs

½ a mango, (approx. 100g) peeled and diced

½ an avocado, peeled and diced

40g rocket

lemon juice

chilli flakes

sea salt and freshly ground black pepper

Heat the oil in a frying pan. Add the chicken and dried herbs and sauté for 4 to 5 minutes, until cooked.

Serve the chicken with the mango, avocado and rocket. Drizzle with a little lemon juice, and sprinkle over a pinch of chilli flakes, salt and pepper.

brown rice bowl

{Serves 2}

It's lovely to have something different for breakfast once in a while. Rice is a good source of fibre and offers a little protein as well as the essential minerals manganese and magnesium. It's also a naturally gluten-free grain.

1 x 250g packet of cooked brown rice (or 100g uncooked brown rice)

150g mushrooms, sliced

2 tablespoons olive oil

sea salt and freshly ground black pepper

400g spinach

1 clove of garlic, crushed

2 eggs

½ an avocado, peeled and sliced

juice of ½ a lemon

If using uncooked rice, cook it according to the packet instructions. Put a large pan of water on to boil, ready to poach your eggs later.

Fry the mushrooms in 1 tablespoon of the olive oil in a large sauté pan or frying pan and season well with salt and pepper. Don't crowd the pan. Fry until golden, then remove the mushrooms from the pan.

Using the same pan, sauté the spinach with another tablespoon of olive oil and the crushed garlic (you may need to add the spinach a handful at a time). It's nicest if the spinach is just wilted, and that way it doesn't go too soggy.

Poach the eggs and season them with a little salt and pepper.

If using a packet of pre-cooked rice, heat this now.

Divide everything between two bowls, including the avocado, and serve warm, dressed with the lemon juice.

tip: You can replace the rice with quinoa, buckwheat, pearl barley or puy lentils.

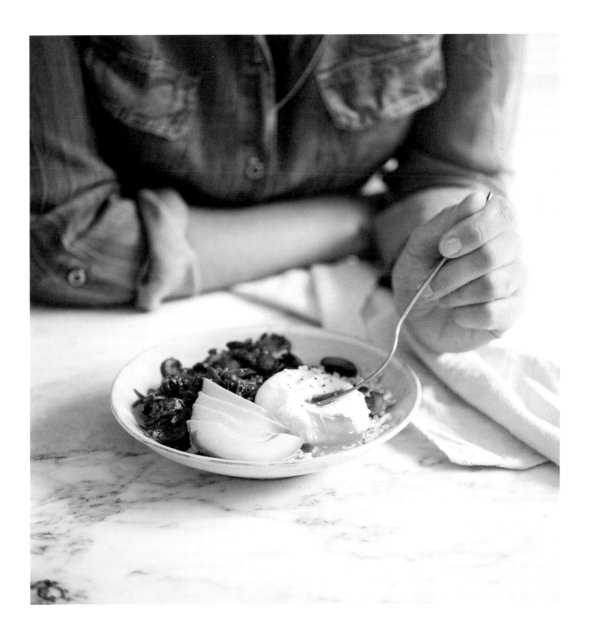

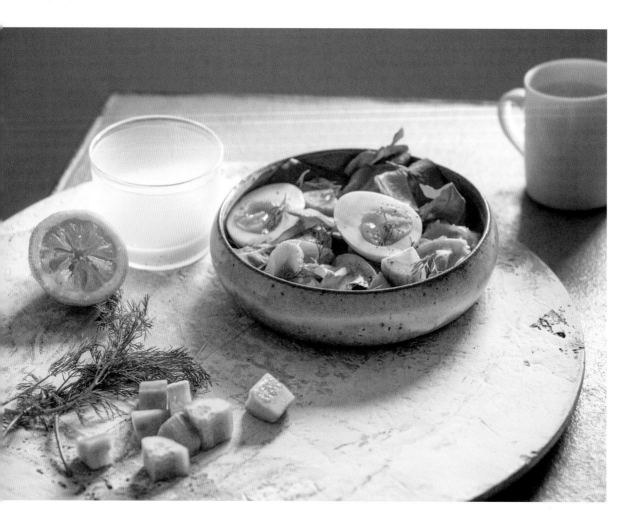

salmon breakfast bowl

{Serves 2}

A fresh take on traditional smoked salmon and scrambled eggs, with the added bonus of two portions of vegetables. This can be made the night before if time is short, and of course is just as good at lunch or supper.

2 large eggs

4 slices of smoked salmon (approx. 80g)

¼ of a cucumber, chopped

½ a head of lettuce, leaves torn

For the dressing

juice of 1 lemon

1 tablespoon apple cider vinegar

1 teaspoon honey

½ teaspoon Dijon mustard

a pinch of sea salt

freshly ground black pepper

1 tablespoon chopped fresh dill (or ½ teaspoon of dried)

Put the eggs into a pan of cold water and bring to the boil. Boil the eggs for 6 to 7 minutes, then immediately dunk them into cold water. Peel and slice in half.

To make the dressing, whisk everything together – this can be done ahead of time, but add the chopped dill at the last moment.

Arrange the smoked salmon, cucumber, lettuce and boiled eggs in a bowl and drizzle over the lemony dill dressing.

mini frittatas

Frittatas have been a staple breakfast for me over the years, as they are a great way to pack in the all-important vegetables that we know we need to eat every day. These 'mini' versions made in a muffin tray make great finger foods, and so are a brilliant option for toddlers. Naturally you can use any vegetables that you have or like. We pile them up on a plate, and Willow loves that we all take it in turns to select one and eat them together. They freeze well too.

{Makes 12}

olive oil, for greasing

4 mushrooms, finely chopped

4 cherry tomatoes, finely chopped

2 baby potatoes (approx. 85g), boiled and finely chopped

a pinch of mixed dried herbs

sea salt and freshly ground black pepper

8 large eggs, whisked

Preheat the oven to 200°C/180°C fan. Grease a muffin tin with olive oil (I use a piece of kitchen paper to spread the oil evenly around the holes).

Mix the vegetables and herbs together in a bowl, season well with salt and pepper, then distribute between the muffin holes. Pour over the whisked egg, being careful to avoid it spilling over the edges.

Bake in the oven for 12 to 15 minutes, or until cooked through.

Allow to cool, then use a knife to loosen the edges of the frittatas, lift them out and serve immediately.

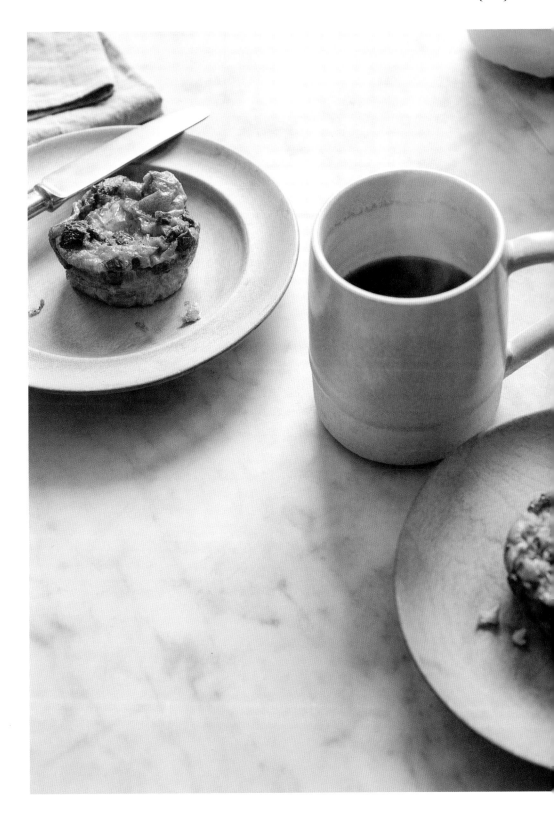

fried egg flatbreads with black beans, avocado & cashew cream

My dream breakfast on a lazy weekend or holiday. You can use sour cream or crème fraîche if you prefer, or omit the eggs if you are vegan.

{Serves 2}

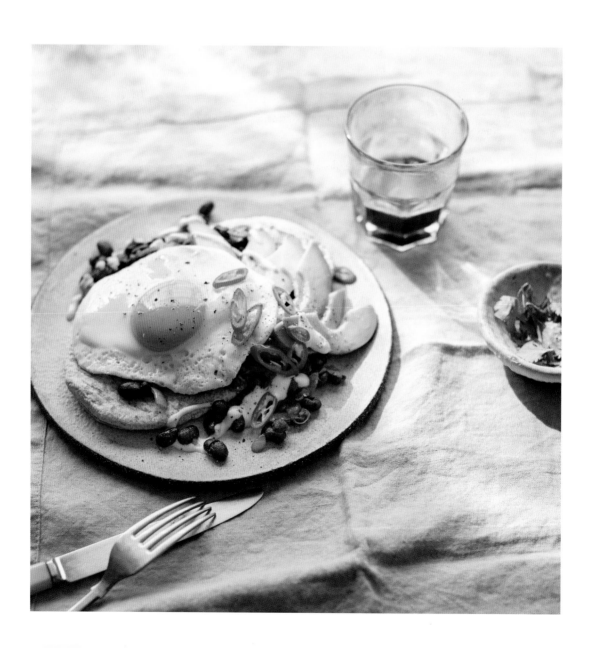

1 tablespoon olive oil

½ an onion, peeled and finely diced

1 clove of garlic, peeled and crushed

½ teaspoon sea salt

¼ teaspoon paprika

1 x 400g tin of black beans, drained and rinsed

2 eggs

2 pitta breads or Yoghurt Flatbreads (see page 109)

1 avocado, peeled and sliced

fresh coriander leaves

fresh chilli or dried chilli flakes (optional)

For the cashew cream

½ cup (90g) of whole raw cashews

1 tablespoon freshly squeezed lemon juice

1 teaspoon apple cider vinegar

¼ teaspoon sea salt

3–4 tablespoons water

First make the cashew cream. Put the cashews into a bowl and pour over at least 3 cups (750ml) of boiling water. Leave to soak at room temperature for 15 minutes, then drain the cashews in a colander or sieve, and rinse.

Place the soaked cashews in the pitcher of a high-speed blender along with the lemon juice, vinegar, salt and 3 tablespoons of water. Purée on maximum speed until the mixture is completely smooth, and has the consistency of double cream. You may need to add the extra tablespoon of water. Taste and add more salt if needed, then set aside.

Heat a pan on a medium heat, then add the olive oil. Once warm, add the onion and garlic. Add the salt and stir often, to soften the onions. Don't let them burn.

Once soft, add the paprika and the drained black beans. Cook for another few minutes to warm the beans. Reduce the heat to low.

Meanwhile, fry the eggs and put the pitta bread or yoghurt flatbreads in to toast.

When ready to serve, pile half the beans on top of each toasted pitta, and tumble over some sliced avocado. Drizzle each one with some cashew cream, and add a fried egg.

Finally, sprinkle with fresh coriander leaves and finely chopped fresh chilli or chilli flakes.

tip: Any leftover cashew cream can be stored in a jar in the fridge for 3 to 4 days. It can also be frozen.

LUNCH

2}

instant tomato & cannellini bean soup

(vegan)

{Serves 3}

This is an 'instant' soup. Simply blend the raw ingredients together in a decent blender, and it's ready. No cooking required. With this particular one, you can even make it when the fridge is looking decidedly bare, as it is mainly composed of tinned ingredients. Enjoy it gently warmed through, or chilled like a gazpacho. If you have any left over, it freezes well (although heat it through thoroughly before serving).

2 x 400g tins of good-quality chopped tomatoes, plus ½ a tin (200ml) of cold water to rinse them out

1 x 400g tin or jar of cannellini beans, drained and rinsed

1 spring onion, roughly chopped

2 tablespoons extra virgin olive oil, plus extra to drizzle

½ teaspoon sea salt

1 tablespoon cider vinegar

a handful of fresh basil leaves

freshly ground black pepper

Put all the ingredients (including the cold water) into the blender, and blend until completely smooth. Add a little more water to adjust the consistency if needed. Either chill or heat to serve.

Serve with a good grind of black pepper and a drizzle of olive oil.

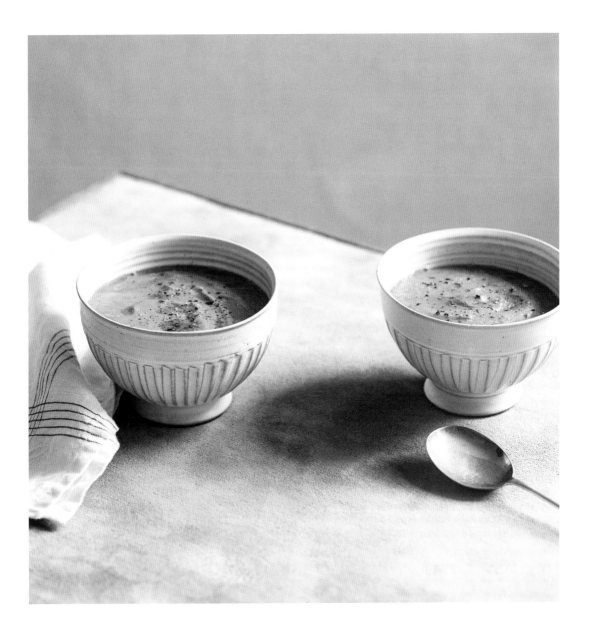

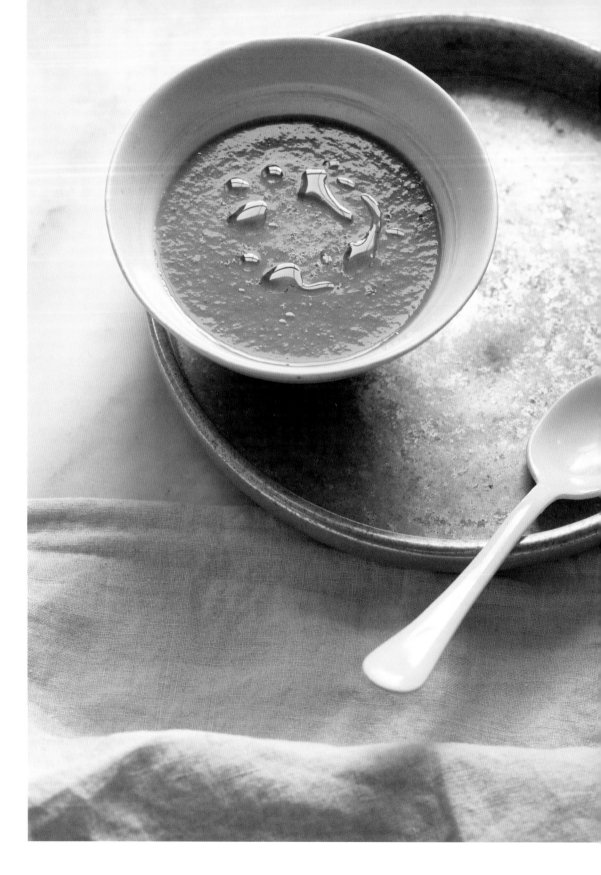

instant
watercress
& avocado
soup
(vegan)

{Serves 1}

This soup is the most beautiful, verdant green, packed with antioxidants and vitamins, and is surprisingly filling (because of the avocado). The seeds are essential to add protein to the meal, so don't skip those (even though we forgot to add them in this photo!). Alternatively, add cooked chicken or fish if you have some.

1 spring onion,
roughly chopped

½ a small ripe avocado

½ teaspoon bouillon
powder, made up to 300ml
with just-boiled water
(or 300ml hot stock)

50g watercress (a very
large handful)

sea salt and freshly
ground black pepper

a small grating of nutmeg,
to serve (optional)

2 tablespoons mixed seeds

Blend all the ingredients together, apart from the nutmeg and seeds (make sure the lid is firmly attached to your blender to avoid the hot liquid spraying out), then taste and adjust the seasoning if necessary.

Grate a little fresh nutmeg on top, if using, and sprinkle with the seeds.

soup for the soul

{Serves 4}

My plant-based version of the classic chicken and lemon soup. Here, chickpeas provide the protein and give a deliciously thick and creamy texture. It will thicken in the fridge, so just warm it up and stir well, to serve. The lemon lends a refreshing lift, perfect for a chilly summer or early autumn evening.

1 x 400g tin of chickpeas, drained and rinsed

olive oil

sea salt and freshly ground black pepper

1 onion, peeled and roughly chopped

1 clove of garlic, peeled and roughly chopped

1 carrot, peeled and roughly chopped

1 litre chicken or vegetable stock (I use half and half)

zest and juice of 1 lemon

To serve

roasted chickpeas* (optional)

a pinch of chilli flakes (optional)

chopped fresh parsley

In a large non-stick saucepan, sauté the onions and garlic in about 1 tablespoon of olive oil for 10 to 15 minutes, until soft. Do not let them brown.

Add the carrots and cook for a further 5 to 10 minutes, stirring occasionally to prevent the vegetables catching. Add a little water if needed.

Add the chickpeas, mix well, then pour over the stock. Bring to the boil, then reduce to a simmer for 10 minutes.

Add the lemon zest and juice, and blend until smooth – either cool for 10 to 15 minutes and blend with a stick blender, or cool completely if using a blender or food processor.

Reheat gently or cool before serving as desired. Serve sprinkled with the roasted chickpeas, chilli flakes, if using, and chopped parsley.

*
tip: To make roasted chickpeas, drain and rinse a tin of chickpeas. Drizzle with a little olive oil (about 2 teaspoons), sprinkle with salt and pepper and roast on a small baking tray for 10 to 20 minutes in a preheated oven (200°C/180°C fan).

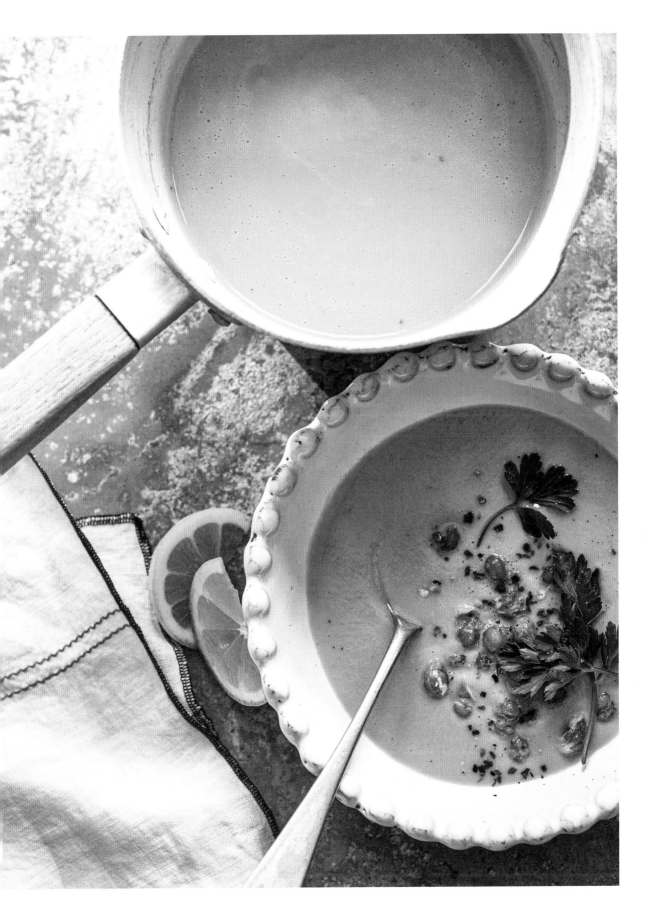

coconut & chicken soup with courgette noodles

{Serves 3}

This is best served straight away, as courgette noodles can go a bit mushy. But if you want to save a portion for another day, add the courgette and greens when serving.

1 x 400ml tin of light coconut milk

300ml vegetable or chicken stock (bouillon is good)

1cm fresh ginger, peeled and cut into thin slices

½ teaspoon fish sauce

1 teaspoon honey

2 skinless chicken breasts, cut into chunks (approx. 2.5cm)

150g mushrooms, sliced

1 large courgette, cut into noodles, using a spiralizer, julienne peeler or vegetable peeler

2 handfuls of leafy greens, such as kale or spinach

a handful of fresh coriander, roughly chopped

¼ teaspoon dried chilli flakes

1 lime: juice of ½ and remaining half cut into 3 wedges, to serve

Put the coconut milk into a pan with the stock, ginger, fish sauce and honey. Bring to the boil.

Add the chicken and the mushrooms and simmer gently for 6 minutes. Add the courgette noodles and leafy greens and cook for a further 2 minutes. Check that the chicken is cooked through. Finish with chopped coriander, the chilli flakes and the lime juice, and serve with wedges of lime.

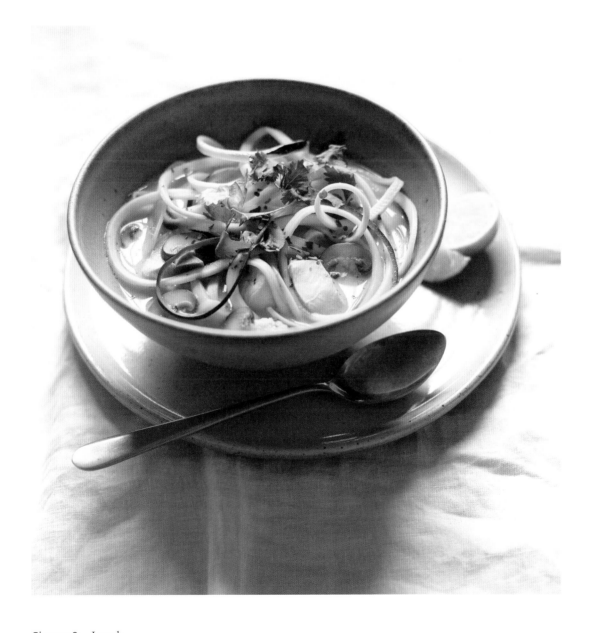

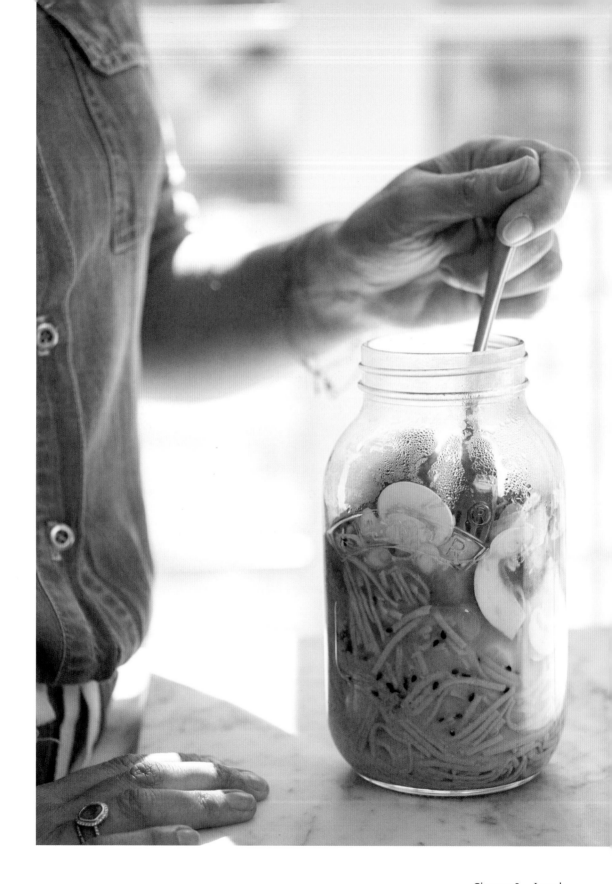

miso
& broccoli
'noodle pot'
(vegan)

{Serves 2}

Miso paste is made from fermented soybeans and is rich in nutrients, protein and beneficial bacteria. In Japan, miso soup is a favoured breakfast, and I could happily eat this noodle pot for breakfast too. The vegetables remain lovely and crunchy and I find the umami flavour really soothing and satisfying. This is a light but heavenly meal.

2 x 85g bundles of buckwheat noodles

2 teaspoons sesame oil

1 teaspoon grated fresh ginger

2 teaspoons miso paste

1 heaped teaspoon vegetable bouillon

1 tablespoon tahini

1 tablespoon tamari

sea salt and freshly ground black pepper

8 mushrooms, sliced

1 spring onion, sliced

¼ of a head of broccoli, cut into very small florets

1 tablespoon sesame seeds

Cook the noodles according to the packet instructions, then drain well, run under cold water and drain again. Toss with the sesame oil, then divide between two resealable 750ml glass jars.

Divide the ginger, miso, bouillon, tahini and tamari between the jars. Season with salt and pepper. Add the mushrooms, spring onions, broccoli and sesame seeds, and keep in the fridge until ready to eat.

When ready to serve, pour in boiling water to reach the top of the jar (about 375ml), then put the lid back on and leave to sit for 2 minutes. Stir well and serve.

vegetable minestrone

{Serves 6}

This is thick, rich and bursting with flavour as well as colourful, microbe-friendly vegetables and plant proteins. Authentic minestrone soup usually has pasta, rice or potatoes, but I find the beans are enough to make it filling and chunky. It can be frozen too.

For the base

1 clove of garlic, peeled

½ **an onion**, peeled and cut into quarters

1 **celery stalk**, cut into chunks

1 **large carrot**, peeled and cut into chunks

1 tablespoon olive oil

For the soup

1 **large courgette**, cut into 1cm dice

1 **large carrot**, peeled and cut into 1cm dice

1 x 400g **tin of cannellini beans**, drained and rinsed

1 x 400g **tin of plum tomatoes**

800ml **stock**, chicken or vegetable

sea salt and freshly ground black pepper

a large handful of seasonal greens, such as kale, cavolo nero or Swiss chard, chopped

Place all the ingredients for the base, except for the olive oil, in a food processor and pulse until finely chopped.

Put the olive oil into a large heavy-based saucepan and tip in the blitzed vegetables. Cook without browning over a gentle heat for 10 minutes, stirring occasionally.

Add the courgette, carrot, cannellini beans, tinned tomatoes and stock. Use a wooden spoon to break up the tomatoes. Season well with salt and pepper. Cover with a lid and bring to the boil, then reduce the heat and cook for 30 minutes.

Once the vegetables are soft, add the chopped seasonal greens and cook for a further 5 minutes, until cooked to your liking.

Check and adjust the seasoning, and serve.

tip: If you prefer a smoother soup, then this is easy to blend. I like to swirl a little pesto on top for a pop of flavour.

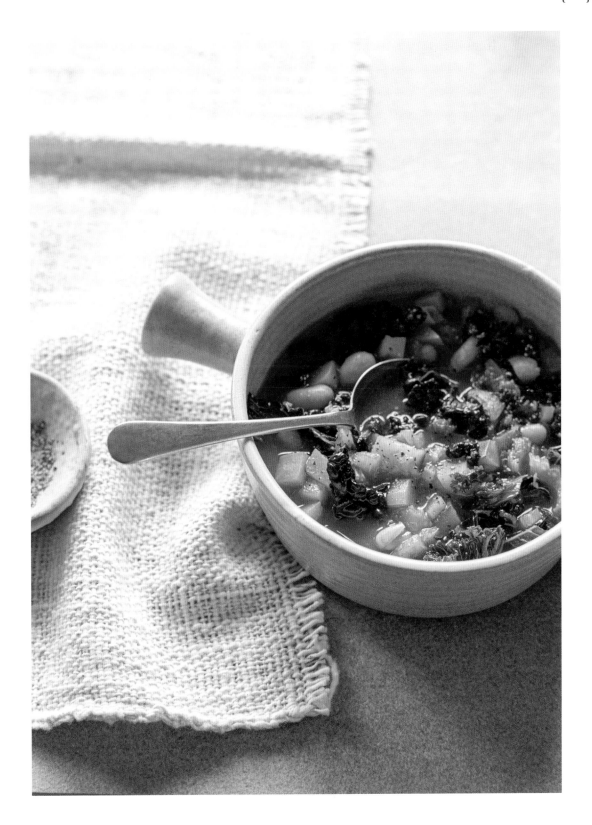

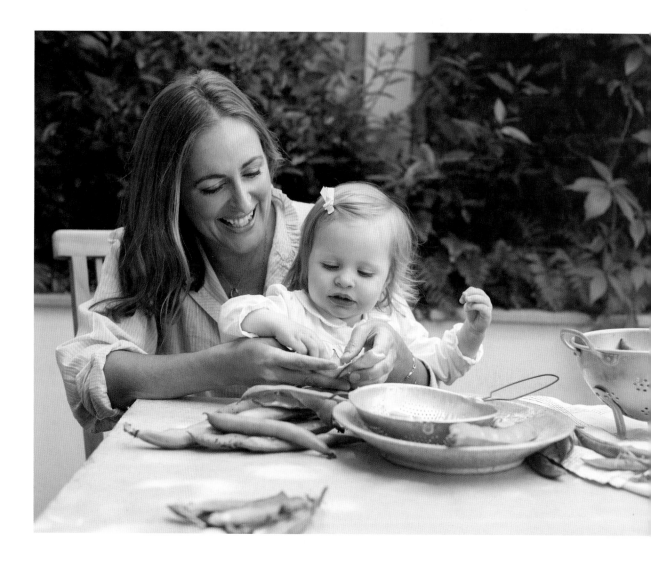

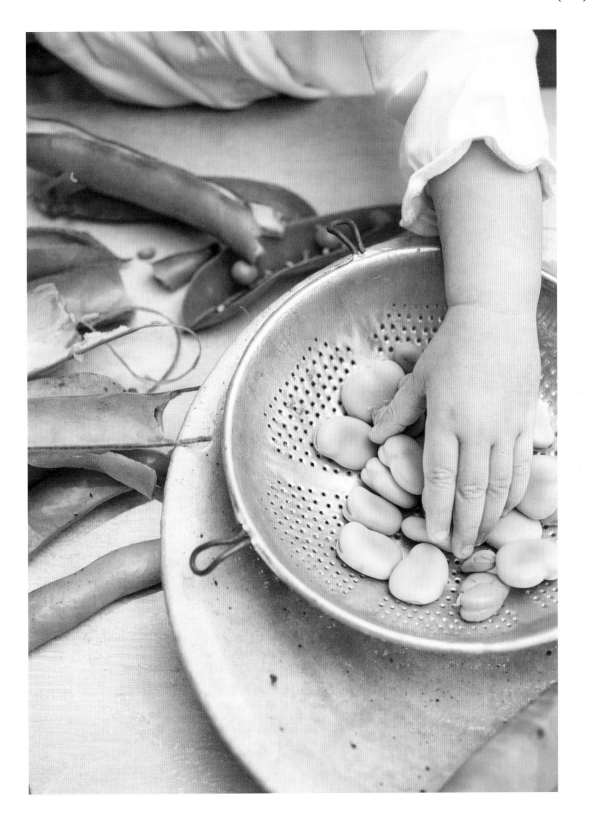

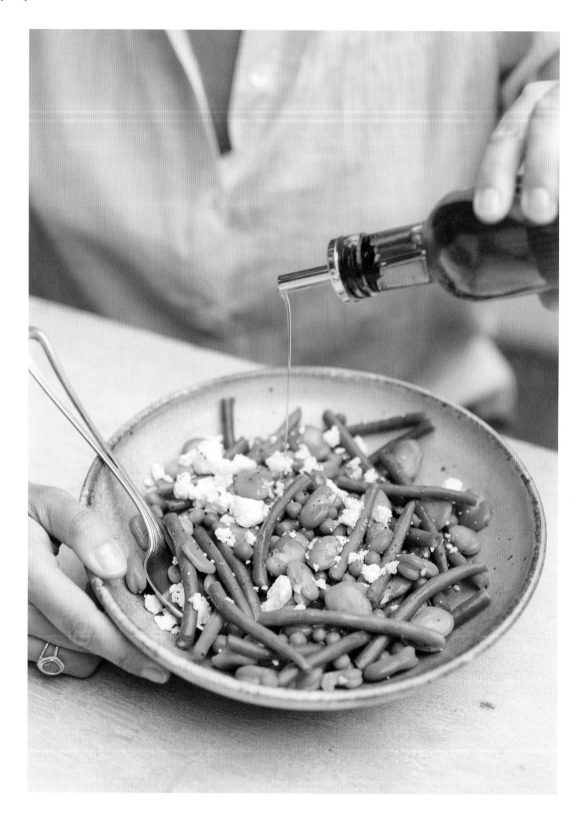

cheat's green bean salad

{Serves 2}

This may be a 'cheat' recipe, but it's one that I find myself turning to again and again, especially when busy. The joy of it lies in the fact that there is no vegetable prep required, as they all come straight from the freezer. But don't let that worry you – unrefined frozen foods are often just as good as (sometimes even better than) their fresh counterparts, because they are frozen so soon after picking that they retain plenty of nutrients. This is also delicious cold the next day.

2 cups frozen baby broad beans (310g)

2 cups frozen green beans (200g)

2 cups frozen peas (250g)

50g feta

olive oil

sea salt and freshly ground black pepper

In a large steamer, steam the beans for 4 to 5 minutes, adding the peas after 2 minutes, until defrosted and heated through.

Toss into a bowl, crumble over the feta and add a little drizzle of olive oil, plus salt and pepper to taste. Stir well together and serve.

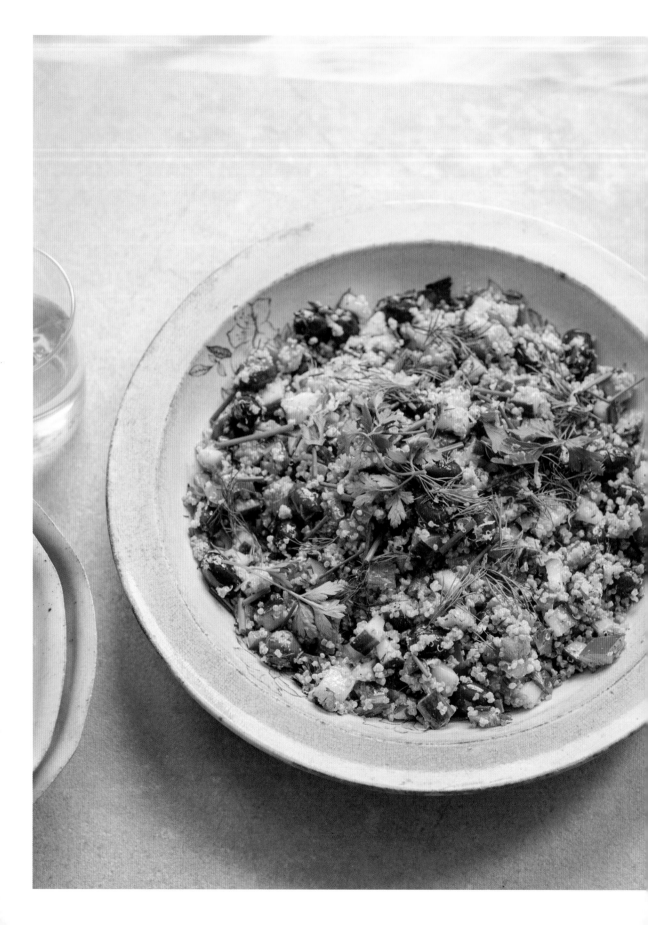

mediterranean quinoa salad

{Serves 4}

Simple, chopped salads like this one are a staple for me. My time-saving tip is to use a packet of pre-cooked quinoa if you don't have time to cook the quinoa from scratch. This is a lovely meal – just as it is, or you can serve it with fish or chicken if feeding a crowd.

1 cucumber, diced

2 red peppers, deseeded and diced

200g pitted black olives

1 bunch of a mix of whatever fresh herbs you have (such as parsley, dill, chives, basil, coriander – and rocket also works)

zest and juice of 1 lemon

1 tablespoon ground almonds

4 tablespoons extra virgin olive oil

sea salt and freshly ground black pepper

250g cooked quinoa*

Mix all the ingredients together in a bowl, and store covered in the fridge.

This keeps well, and actually tastes better the next day.

*
tip: See page 100 for instructions on cooking quinoa from dried.

poached salmon with preserved lemon & herb quinoa

{Serves 2}

I think lemon might just be my favourite ingredient. Many meals can be positively invigorated with a squeeze of juice or a little zest. Preserved lemons are even more enriching, and can easily be made by pickling whole lemons in salt and lemon juice for 4 weeks (there are many online recipes for this). It leaves the deep fragrance of the peel without the tartness. If you haven't tried them, this recipe is a great place to start. Serve with some salad or steamed greens.

100g quinoa or 250g pre-cooked quinoa

2 wild salmon fillets

fresh dill/parsley stalks (optional)

sea salt and freshly ground black pepper

For the dressing

1 tablespoon each, finely chopped: mint, basil, chives, parsley, dill, spring onion

2 preserved lemons, seeds removed, finely chopped, plus 1 tablespoon of the lemon juice from the jar

1 tablespoon white wine vinegar

4 tablespoons olive oil

1 teaspoon maple syrup or honey

If cooking the quinoa from scratch: place the rinsed quinoa in a pan, cover with roughly the same amount of water and a generous pinch of salt then bring to the boil. Reduce to a simmer and cook, uncovered, for 10 minutes, until the water is almost totally absorbed but the quinoa still has a little bite. Turn off the heat, put the lid back on and leave to sit for another 10 minutes to steam and finish cooking.

Put the salmon into a shallow frying pan with a lid, and add just enough cold water to cover it. Add some flavours (e.g. lemon zest, dill and parsley stalks, salt and pepper) to the water if you like. Bring to the boil, simmer for 2 minutes, then remove from the heat and allow the salmon to sit in the hot water until cooked and light pink in the middle. Remove from the pan and flake with a fork.

To make the dressing, put all the chopped herbs into a bowl with the chopped preserved lemons, a little lemon juice from their jar, the white wine vinegar, olive oil, your choice of sweetener, and salt and pepper to taste, and stir it together well.

Stir 2 tablespoons of the herby dressing through the warm quinoa. Serve the flaked salmon on top of the quinoa and drizzle the rest of the dressing on top. Check and adjust the seasoning, and serve.

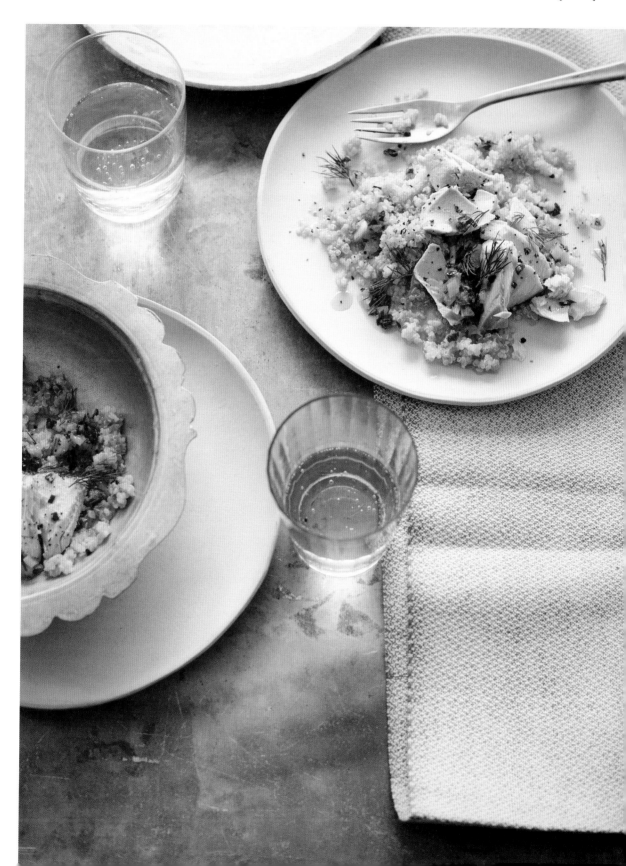

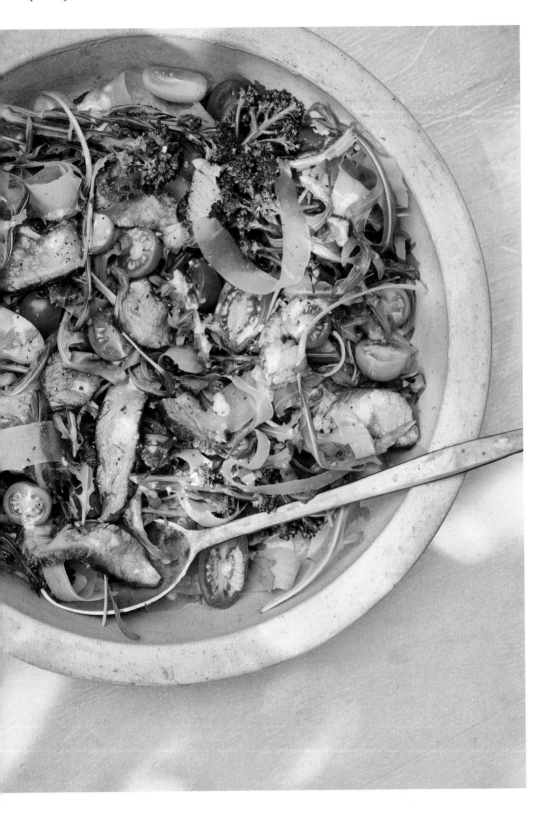

beef & rocket salad with creamy horseradish

{Serves 2}

This salad is an easy way to use up any leftover roast beef if you have roasted a joint, but if not, you could use ready-cooked beef from a supermarket or thinly sliced strips of pan-fried steak. Steak and rocket go wonderfully well with horseradish in a sandwich but I wanted a lighter version and more vegetables, so this simple salad happened and the dressing is a firm favourite now.

1 small head of broccoli, or a handful of sprouting broccoli, cut into bite-size florets

a few slices (around 100–150g) of cold, cooked beef*

1 bag of rocket (approx. 90g)

1 large carrot, peeled, then, using the peeler, shaved into ribbons

10 cherry tomatoes, halved

sourdough toast, to serve (optional)

For the dressing

2 tablespoons extra virgin olive oil

1 tablespoon creamed horseradish

1 tablespoon apple cider vinegar

a generous pinch of sea salt

Steam (or boil) the broccoli florets for 3 to 4 minutes, until they are a bright green. Drain and allow to cool.

If using leftover beef, you might wish to warm it gently through in the oven or microwave, to bring it back to life before using.

Whisk together all the dressing ingredients until well combined and creamy.

Combine all the ingredients in a big bowl and toss with the dressing, so it thoroughly coats everything. Pile on to a plate and serve, perhaps with a slice or two of sourdough toast drizzled with olive oil on the side.

*
tip: I often use leftovers from the Slow-cooked Beef Brisket recipe on page 206 to make this salad.

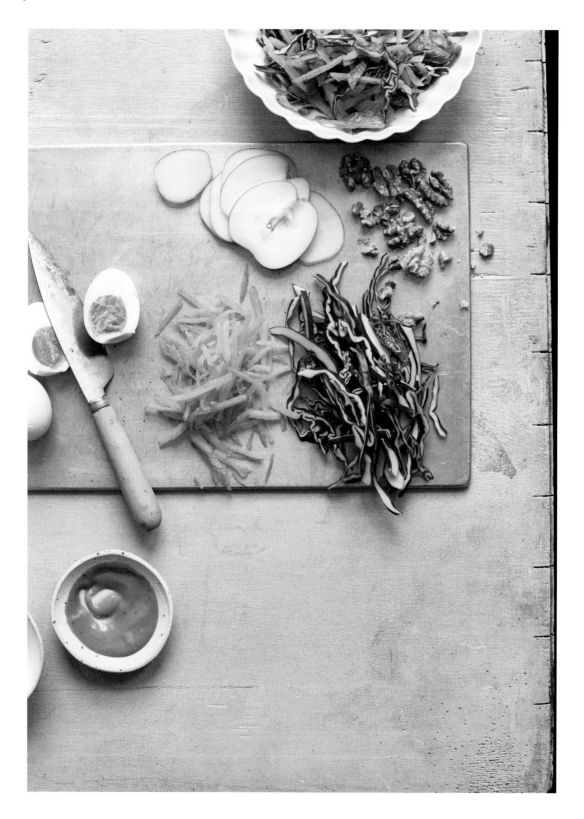

waldorf slaw with balsamic tahini dressing

{Serves 2}

This riff on a Waldorf salad contains a variety of colourful vegetables (providing fibre, vitamins and beneficial phytonutrients), eggs (for protein) and walnuts (for healthy fats and various essential minerals), as well as chopped apples for tang and sweetness and a deliciously creamy balsamic tahini dressing to replace the traditional mayonnaise. Omit the eggs and double the amount of chopped walnuts if you'd like to keep it plant-based.

2 large handfuls of spinach, chopped

1 large carrot, peeled and grated

¼ of a red cabbage, finely chopped

½ an apple, finely sliced

2 hard-boiled eggs, roughly chopped

30g walnuts, toasted and roughly chopped

sea salt and freshly ground black pepper

For the dressing

2 tablespoons tahini

1 tablespoon balsamic vinegar

1 teaspoon maple syrup

¼ teaspoon water

¼ teaspoon sea salt

a grind of black pepper

Whisk all the ingredients for the dressing together in a large mixing bowl until well combined. Add the salad ingredients directly to the bowl.

Toss together and check the seasoning.

tip: If you have a food processor, this salad is very quick to make by using the grater setting for the vegetables or apple.

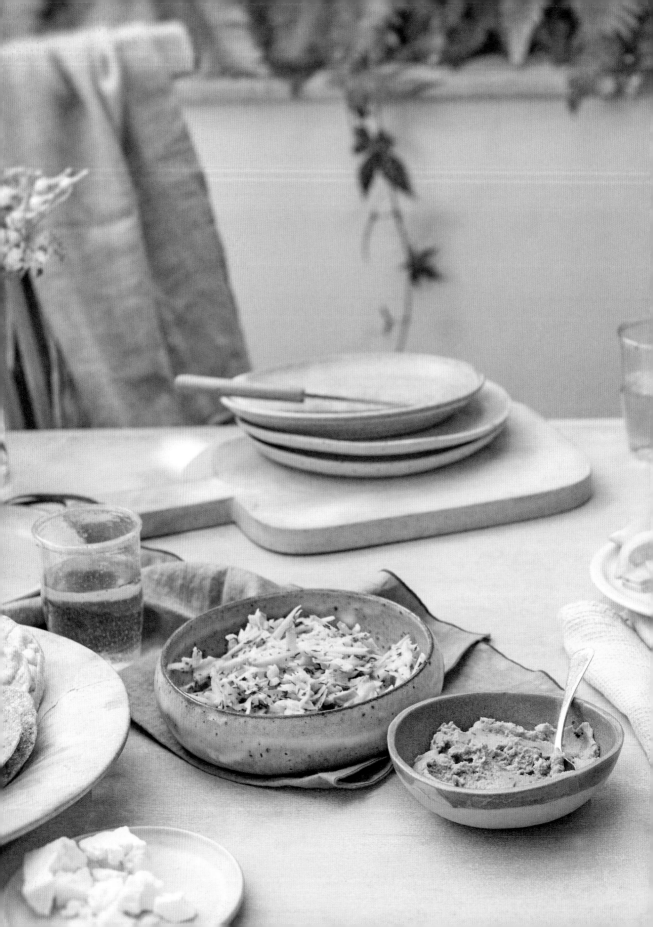

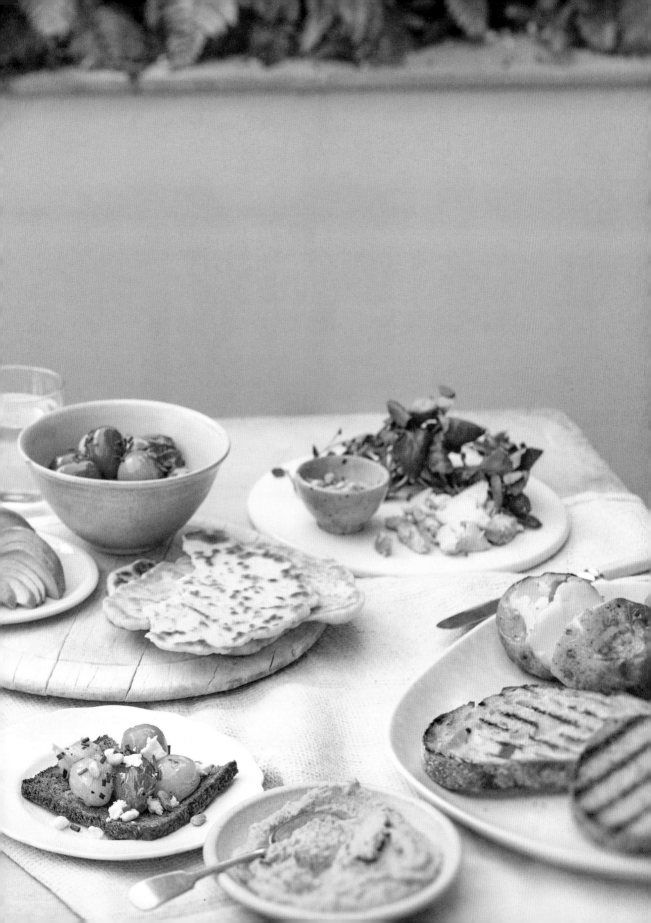

hero
toppings

We all have days when making a full meal from scratch just isn't possible. So for these occasions I started to think up some 'hero toppings' that could be added to toast, or flatbreads, baked potatoes or crackers, to enhance their nutrition and make sure that we are still eating some important nutrients alongside the carbohydrate staples. Admittedly they may take a little more time than simply spreading butter, but these simple additions really can help us feel and see a difference in our energy and vitality. So, this section is for the tired and time-poor – you can still have your toast and eat it! Just be savy with what you put on top.

'Bases' to choose from:

- Wholemeal pitta bread
- Yoghurt flatbreads (see opposite)
- Toasted rye/sourdough/GF bread
- Jacket potatoes
- rice cakes/corn cakes/oat cakes
- Lettuce 'cups'
- Corn/wholemeal tortilla wraps
- Cooked pasta

yoghurt flatbreads

I have been making these flatbreads for many years. I wish I could say I invented this recipe, but alas, it has been around for a long time and there are many versions if you google 'yoghurt flatbreads'. I have tried and tested many different flavours, but when my daughter started to be able to chew, I pulled this recipe right back to these simple ingredients, avoiding the salt in particular, so that she could enjoy them. They couldn't be easier to make and are a staple in my home. I make a batch most weeks and use them as a carrier for lots of wonderfully tasty toppings. They make excellent pizza bases, are delicious dipped into curries or soups, but most of all, I use them for the following 'hero toppings'.

{Makes 4}

150g self-raising flour
(I use Doves Farm,
Gluten Free), plus a little
extra to dust surfaces
and hands

125g unsweetened,
natural yoghurt

olive oil

Mix the flour and yoghurt together in a bowl to form a dough. Use your hands to pull it together – you might need a little extra flour, as the mixture can be quite sticky.

Sprinkle a little flour on a board, and flour your hands too. Split the dough into 4 pieces.

Flatten each out to about ½cm thick or less – I like them to be as thin as possible. You can use a rolling pin, but I just use my hands and keep turning to keep a nice round shape.

Heat a little olive oil (around 1 teaspoon per flatbread) in a frying pan on a medium-high heat and fry the flatbreads one by one for about a minute on each side. After each one, I wipe the pan clean with a bit of damp kitchen paper and take the pan off the heat so as not to burn the oil.

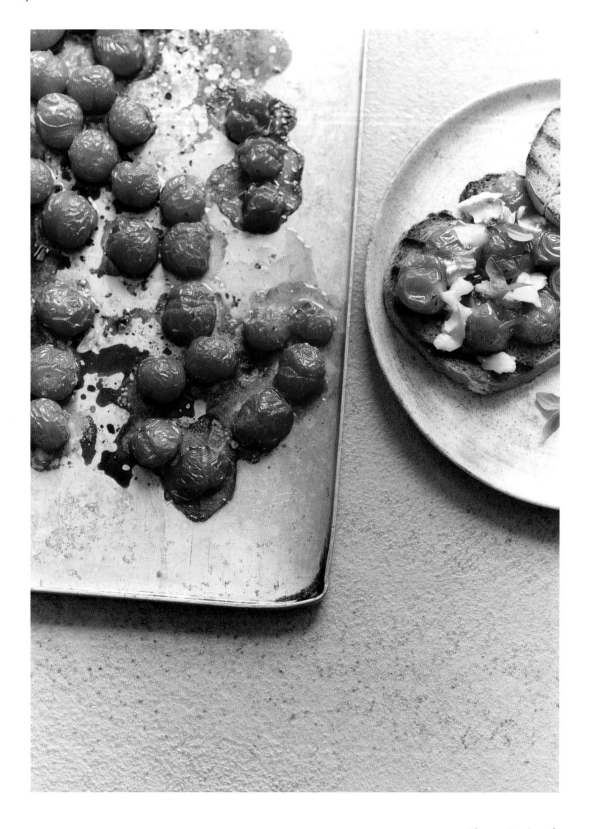

sautéed cherry tomatoes & feta

{Serves 2}

This summery topping is best served warm on toast like a bruschetta, or on toasted pitta or flatbreads. Omit the feta and double the pine nuts for a plant-based alternative. This recipe can easily be doubled to feed more.

15g pine nuts

1 tablespoon olive oil, plus extra for drizzling

300g cherry tomatoes, halved

sea salt and freshly ground black pepper

2x base of your choice (see page 108)

50g feta, crumbled

torn fresh basil leaves or fresh chives (optional)

Heat a non-stick frying pan over a low heat. Add the pine nuts and toast for a few minutes, stirring constantly until lightly golden. Tip on to a plate.

To the same pan, add the oil. Once hot, add the tomatoes, season with salt and pepper, and fry for 2 to 3 minutes, until softening and just starting to collapse, then remove from the heat.

Divide the tomatoes between the base of your choice. Top with the feta and the toasted pine nuts and finish with a drizzle of olive oil, a grind of black pepper and some fresh basil or chives.

celeriac & apple remoulade with smoked trout

{Serves 4}

½ a small celeriac, peeled and coarsely grated

1 Granny Smith apple, grated

150g unsweetened yoghurt

a small bunch of fresh dill, finely chopped

juice of 1 lemon

sea salt and freshly ground black pepper

4 x base of your choice (see page 108)

200g smoked trout, broken into large flakes

Mix the celeriac, apple, yoghurt, dill and lemon juice together. Season well with salt and pepper.

Spread the remoulade over the base of your choice and top with smoked trout.

soya beans & mint

(vegan)

{Serves 4}

350g frozen soya beans

a small bunch of fresh mint, leaves finely chopped

a pinch of chilli flakes

juice of 2 limes

2 tablespoons olive oil

sea salt and freshly ground black pepper

4 x base of your choice (see page 108)

Cook the soya beans in a pan of boiling water for 2 to 3 minutes, until hot through. Drain under cold running water.

Put the beans into a food processor with the mint, chilli flakes, lime juice, olive oil, salt and pepper. Pulse until you have a rough paste. If it is too stiff add a little water.

Garnish with freshly ground black pepper, olive oil and a few small mint leaves.

Apply to the base of your choice.

tip: Smoked salmon works just as well, if you prefer.

flaked salmon, rocket, sliced avocado & mayonnaise

{Serves 2}

2 tablespoons mayonnaise

2 x base of your choice (see page 108)

a handful of watercress
(or rocket)

1 avocado, sliced

100g cooked salmon, flaked

½ a lemon

sea salt and freshly ground black pepper

Spread 1 tablespoon of mayonnaise over the base of your choice. Top with the watercress, then the avocado slices and flaked salmon. Squeeze over the lemon juice and season with salt and pepper.

houmous, red onion, tomatoes, cucumber, rocket & torn basil

(vegan)

{Serves 4}

juice of ½ a lemon

1 tablespoon olive oil

a small bunch of fresh basil leaves, chopped

sea salt and freshly ground black pepper

2 medium tomatoes, sliced (approx. 180g)

½ a cucumber (approx. 150g), halved lengthways, deseeded and sliced on an angle

1 small red onion, finely sliced

4 x base of your choice (see page 108)

40g rocket (or other green leaves)

200g houmous*

Whisk the lemon juice, olive oil, basil, salt and pepper in a medium bowl. Add the tomatoes, cucumber and onion and mix together well.

Top or fill the base of your choice with the leaves, spoonfuls of houmous and finally the dressed salad.

*
tip: See my quick and easy houmous recipe on page 125.

sardine, cucumber & dill pâté

{Serves 2}

Sardines are nutritional powerhouses (high in protein, omega-3 fats, calcium and vitamin D). They are also extremely cheap and readily available. I can sometimes find the flavour overpowering, but this pâté mellows it, and is a great way to include this 'super' food into our diet.

1 tin of sardines in olive oil (approx. 100g), drained (drained weight 70g)

1 generous tablespoon mayonnaise

zest and juice of ½ a lemon

a generous pinch of sea salt and plenty of freshly ground black pepper

1 handful of fresh dill, roughly torn (you can substitute 1 teaspoon dried dill, or a handful of fresh rocket or parsley instead)

10cm piece of cucumber, grated

2 x base of your choice (see page 108)

Place the drained sardine fillets in a mini food processor – no need to remove the skin. Add the mayo, lemon zest, lemon juice, salt and pepper and dill, and blend for a few seconds, until the dill is chopped finely and the sardines are smooth.

Squeeze the grated cucumber to remove some of the water content, then stir this through the sardine pâté.

Scoop the mixture into a small bowl, level the top, and place in the fridge to chill.

Apply to the base of your choice.

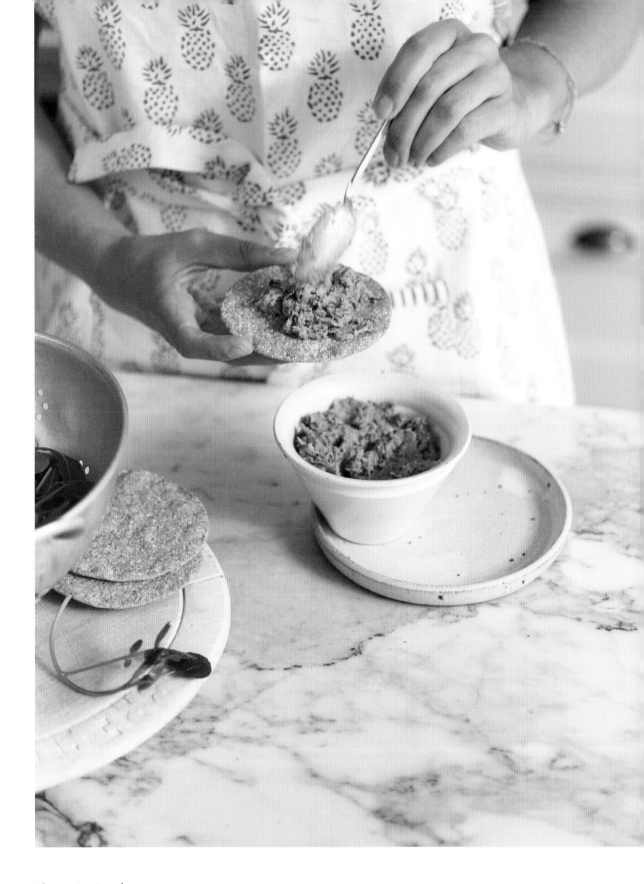

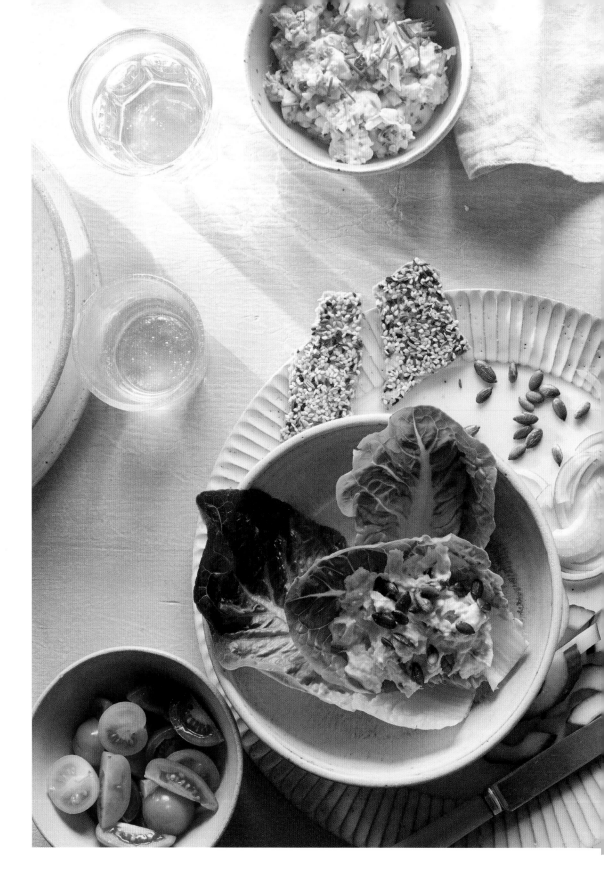

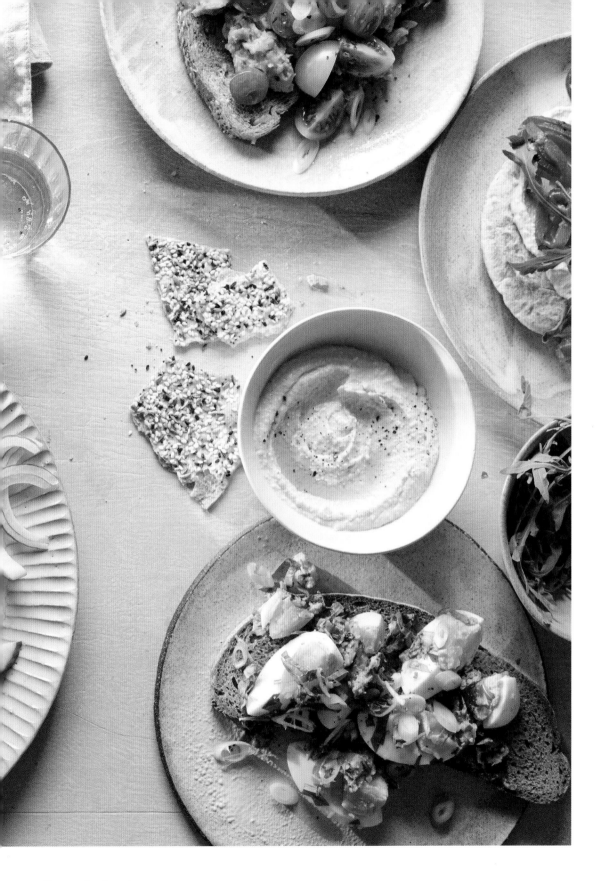

roasted aubergine & butter bean spread
(vegan)

{Serves 4}

I love bean-based dips such as this one, and am rarely without a bowl of it in my fridge. Not only is it great for transforming into lunch at the drop of a hat (just add a big handful of salad leaves and a couple of oatcakes), or for dipping vegetables into as an emergency snack, it is also incredibly cheap and simple to make.

1 aubergine, roughly chopped

2 cloves of garlic, skin on

1 tablespoon olive oil

1 x 400g tin of butter beans, drained and rinsed

juice of ½ a lemon (or 1 tablespoon apple cider vinegar)

1 tablespoon tahini

sea salt and freshly ground black pepper

4 x base of your choice (see page 108)

Preheat the oven to 180°C/160°C fan.

Roast the aubergines and garlic together on a tray, drizzled with the olive oil, until soft and golden (approximately 30 minutes). I usually do this while I have other things cooking in the oven too. Allow to cool slightly, then squeeze the roasted garlic cloves out of their skins.

Blend the roasted aubergine and garlic with the butter beans, lemon juice, tahini and ½ a teaspoon of salt. Add a splash of cold water if it is looking a little bit thick. Taste, adjust the seasoning with salt and pepper and scoop into a covered container.

This will keep for 2 to 3 days in the fridge.

Apply to the base of your choice.

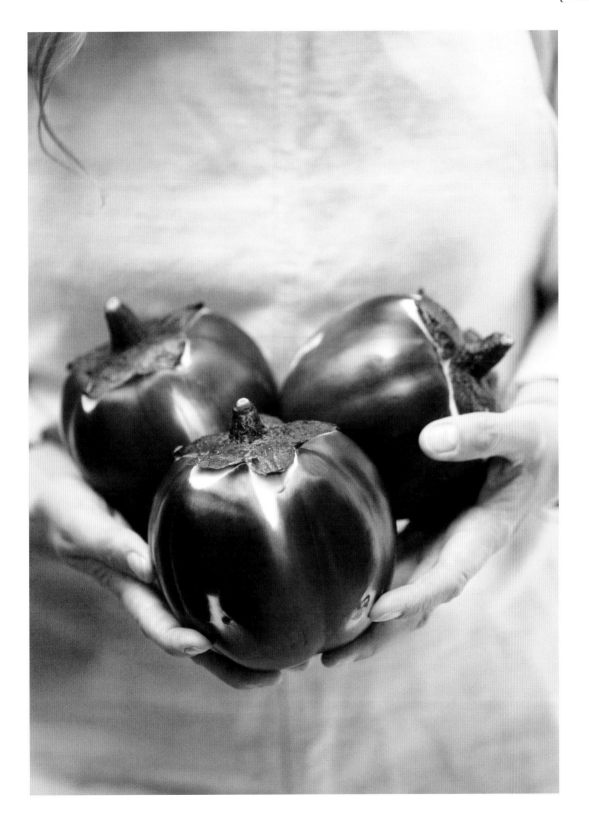

egg mayo

{Serves 4}

6 large eggs

100g unsweetened yoghurt

2 tablespoons finely chopped fresh parsley

2 tablespoons finely chopped fresh chives

3 spring onions, finely chopped

½ teaspoon paprika

sea salt and freshly ground black pepper

4 x base of your choice (see page 108)

Gently drop the eggs into simmering water and boil for 10 minutes. Drain, then place in a large bowl of ice-cold water.

Once cool, peel and mash the eggs. Mix with the yoghurt, herbs, spring onions, paprika, salt and pepper.

This filling will keep in the fridge for 2 days.

Apply to the base of your choice.

green eggs

{Serves 2}

4 medium hard-boiled eggs, peeled

1 medium, ripe avocado, peeled and destoned

1 spring onion, sliced

1 tablespoon apple cider vinegar or white wine vinegar

1 big handful of greens, finely chopped (I like it best with watercress or rocket, but parsley, coriander or spinach would also work well)

sea salt and freshly ground black pepper

2 x base of your choice (see page 108)

In a small bowl, break up the eggs with the back of a fork, then add all the remaining ingredients and mix, mashing the avocado well. You're aiming to get an 'egg mayo' consistency. Taste and season with a generous pinch of salt and plenty of pepper.

Keeps in the fridge for a couple of days if covered. Just mix again before serving.

Apply to the base of your choice.

chicken salad

{Serves 4}

200g cooked chicken breast, shredded

125ml unsweetened yoghurt

zest of 1 lemon

a pinch of chilli flakes

sea salt and freshly ground black pepper

4 x base of your choice (see page 108)

4 small handfuls of rocket or other salad leaves (approx. 40g)

4 medium wholemeal wraps

4 teaspoons pumpkin seeds, toasted

Mix together the chicken, yoghurt, lemon zest, chilli flakes, salt and pepper.

Top the base of your choice with a handful of rocket, then add a quarter of the chicken mix. Sprinkle over the pumpkin seeds. Repeat with the rest of the wraps.

roasted red pepper with houmous, rocket & pumpkin seeds

(vegan)

{Serves 2}

2 x base of your choice (see page 108)

130g houmous*

2 small handfuls of rocket (approx. 25g)

2 roasted red peppers from a jar, finely sliced

olive oil, to drizzle

sea salt and freshly ground black pepper

10g pumpkin seeds, toasted

Spread each base of your choice with half the houmous.

Top with rocket leaves and the sliced red peppers. Drizzle with olive oil and sprinkle with salt and pepper, to taste, and pumpkin seeds to serve.

*
tip: See my quick and easy houmous on page 125.

smashed avocado, rocket, spring onion, cherry tomatoes & chilli flakes

(vegan)

{Serves 2}

1 avocado
a pinch of chilli flakes
juice of 1 lime
1 spring onion, finely chopped
sea salt and freshly ground black pepper
2 x base of your choice (see page 108)
2 small handfuls of rocket (approx. 25g)
8–10 cherry tomatoes, halved
olive oil, to drizzle

Smash the avocado with the back of a fork, then mix with the chilli flakes, 1 tablespoon of lime juice, the spring onion and some salt and pepper.

Spread the avocado over the base of your choice, and top with the rocket and tomatoes. Drizzle with a little extra lime juice and olive oil, to serve.

roasted tomatoes with balsamic goat's cheese & basil

{Serves 2}

400g cherry tomatoes
1 tablespoon olive oil, plus a drizzle to serve
1 tablespoon balsamic vinegar
2 x base of your choice (see page 108)
100g goat's cheese, broken into chunks
a few fresh basil leaves
sea salt and freshly ground black pepper

Heat the oven to 180°C/160°C fan.

Toss the tomatoes with the oil and balsamic. Put them on a tray lined with baking parchment and bake for 25 minutes, until just starting to collapse.

Top the base of your choice with the roasted tomatoes and goat's cheese and return to the grill until the goat's cheese starts to turn golden. Drizzle with oil and sprinkle over some salt and pepper, to taste, and a few torn basil leaves.

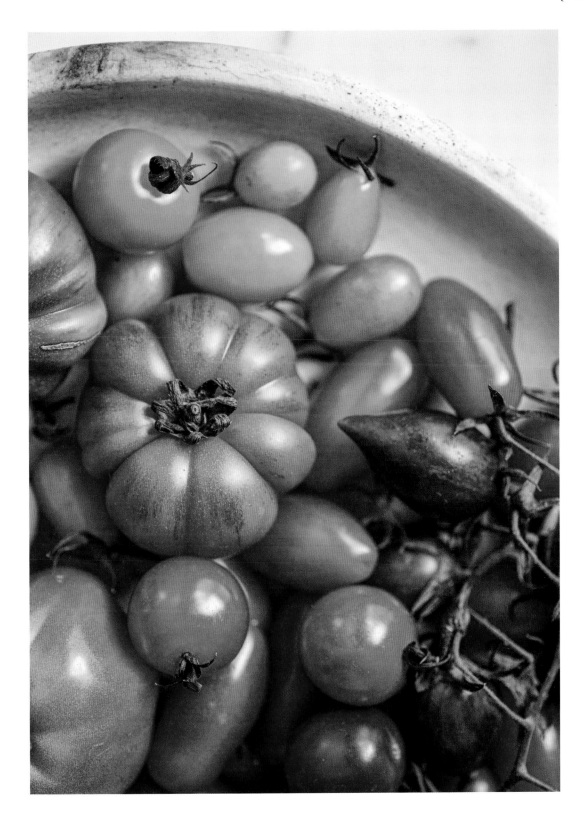

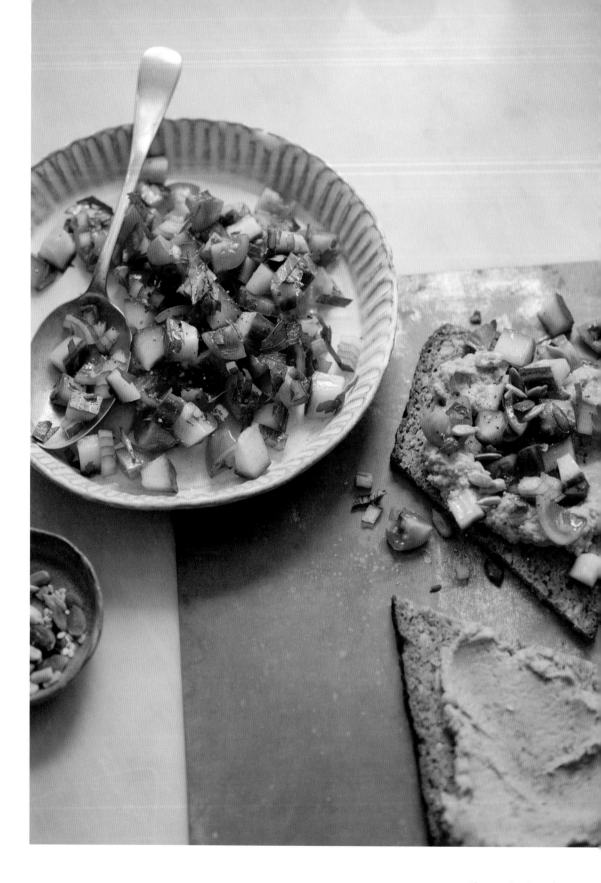

loaded green houmous

{Serves 6}

This is a very quick and easy houmous recipe, and I almost always have some in the fridge. It's much easier to make than you'd imagine and far more economical, too. It lasts for 2 to 3 days.

For the houmous

1 x 400g tin of chickpeas, drained and rinsed

2 tablespoons tahini

1 level teaspoon sea salt

juice of 1 small lemon

2 handfuls of baby leaf spinach

For the salad

1 small red onion, peeled and finely diced

1 cucumber, diced

4 ripe tomatoes, diced

a bunch of fresh parsley, chopped

extra virgin olive oil

optional extras: a handful of seeds, seed sprouts, crumbled feta, olives, chopped sun-dried tomatoes, artichoke hearts

sea salt and freshly ground black pepper

To serve

6 x base of your choice (see page 108)

Blend all the houmous ingredients together in a food processor until smooth, adding extra cold water little by little until you reach your desired consistency. It usually needs 3 to 4 tablespoons or so.

Combine all the salad ingredients together in a bowl, drizzle with a little olive oil, and add a grind of pepper and a pinch of salt.

Spread the green houmous over the base of your choice, using the back of a spoon if necessary. Spoon the salad on top.

pan-fried sardines with chilli, garlic, lemon & parsley

{Serves 2}

Fresh sardines have a much milder flavour then their tinned counterparts, and are worth buying when you find some. Ask the fishmonger to butterfly them. Fillets of fresh mackerel would also work. This is best served warm on toasted bread or flatbreads.

2 tablespoons olive oil

2 cloves of garlic, peeled and crushed

1 red chilli, deseeded and finely chopped

4 butterflied fresh sardine fillets, seasoned

1 lemon, zested and cut into wedges

a small bunch of fresh parsley, finely chopped

2 x base of your choice (see page 108)

Heat the oil in a non-stick frying pan. Add the garlic and chilli and fry for a few seconds, then add the seasoned sardine fillets, skin side down. Fry on a low-medium heat for 3 to 4 minutes, until cooked through. Stir through the lemon zest and parsley.

Serve on the base of your choice, with lemon wedges to squeeze over.

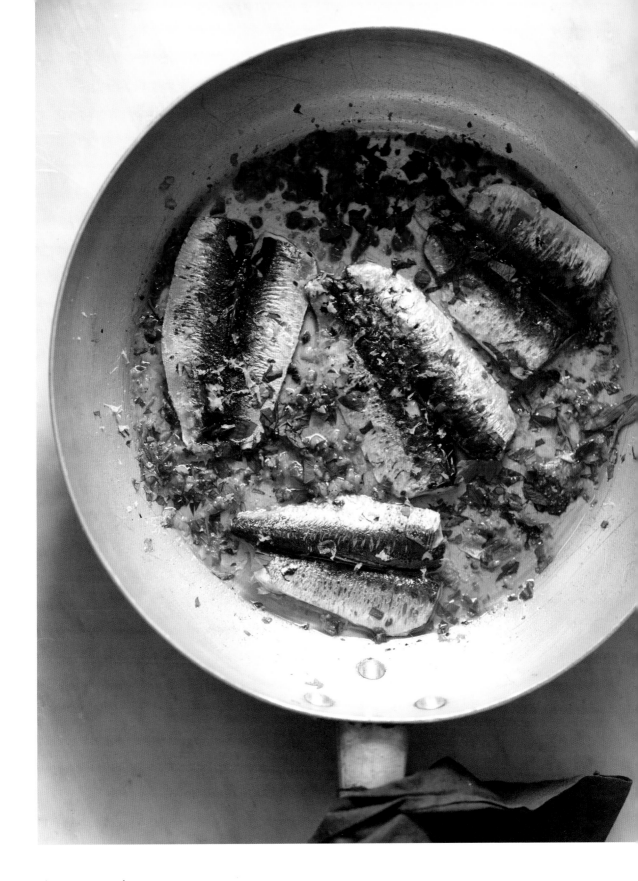

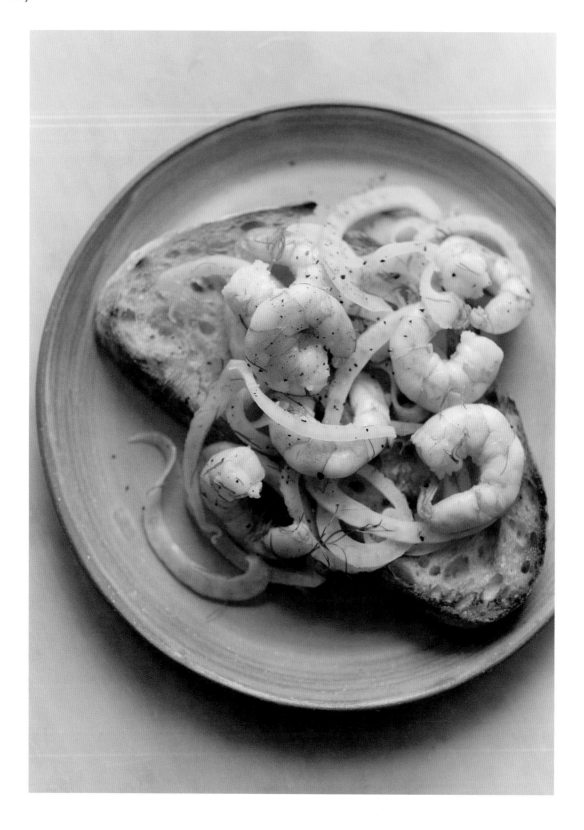

prawns with lemon & fennel salsa

{Serves 2}

Most big supermarkets sell fresh or frozen prawns. Ready-peeled ones are simplest as peeling them can be quite a faff. If using frozen ones, ensure they are thoroughly defrosted first, and consume within 24 hours. I use a mandolin to make this dish as it gets the thinnest slivers of fennel. Otherwise, use a grater.

150g cooked king prawns

juice of 1 lemon

1 small fennel bulb
(approx. 200g),
thinly sliced

a small bunch of fresh dill,
finely chopped

2 tablespoons olive oil

sea salt and freshly
ground black pepper

2 x base of your choice
(see page 108)

Mix all the ingredients together and season with salt and pepper.

Use to fill sandwiches, wraps, lettuce cups or pitta breads, or serve on top of toast.

investment
cooking

Many of us have a limited amount of time to spend in the kitchen preparing food, so we must focus on optimizing the efficiency of that time to create the most nutritious and tasty meals possible. That is where I recommend using the 'investment dishes' concept. When you do have a little more time (perhaps one or two evenings a week, or at the weekend), try cooking a couple of more time-intensive dishes that you can then use to create lots of quick variations for the following few days.

Roasting a chicken is a good example of this, and is something I do most weeks. You will need to invest a couple of hours' cooking time one day to roast the chicken(s), but then you've got cold chicken leftovers that are a ready-to-eat source of protein for the next couple of days, and can form the basis of endless different meals and salads. Three of my favourite examples are given on the following pages, but there really are no 'rules' – use ingredients you enjoy or have in the fridge.

The chicken carcass can also be used (I use a slow cooker for this) to make a chicken stock, which can then make a quick soup or bowl of noodles. If you don't get time to cook a whole chicken from scratch, then I suggest buying a rôtisserie chicken or ready-cooked chicken pieces from a supermarket. The downside of this is that there is usually less choice about the provenance of the bird.

The same 'investment dish' concept can also be applied to roasted vegetables. It takes some time to prepare and roast them, but once cooked, they are a delicious and healthy resource to use for lots more dishes, with very little additional effort.

There are many, many more examples of investment dishes, from ratatouille (see page 151) to big bowls of salad, poached fish to chilli. These are just a few to get you started.

tip: When creating any salads, try to include a selection of different coloured vegetables. 'Eating the rainbow' might sound like a slightly clichéd phrase, but it has good scientific rationale, as each colour found in fresh produce is associated with a different group of nutritional compounds. The more colourful, the better.

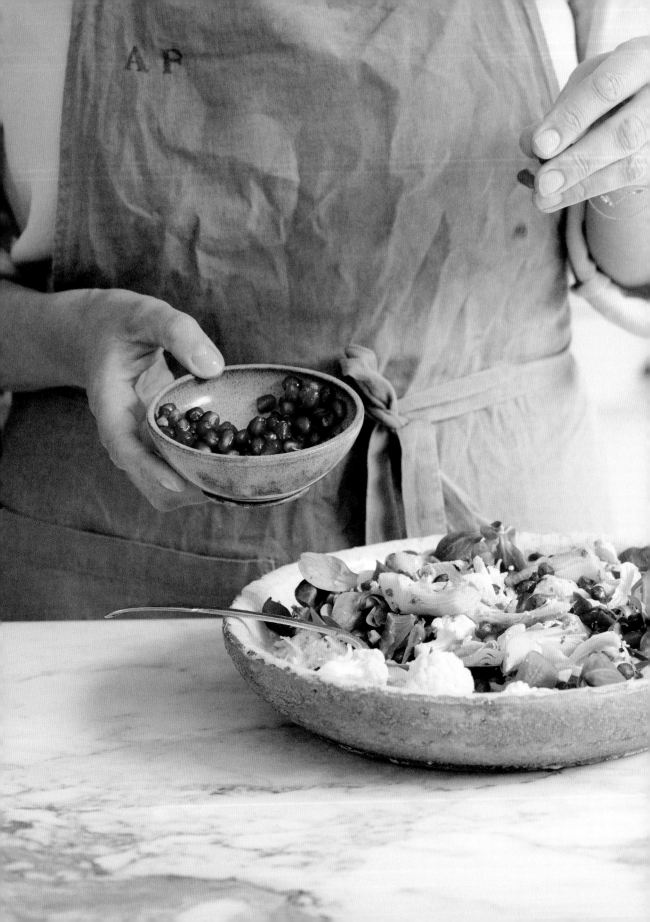

leftover chicken salads

Lentil & Lemon

Rocket & Beetroot

Cauliflower & Pistachio

~

leftover roasted veg salads

Pesto, Brown Rice, Pumpkin Seeds
& Goat's Cheese

Chickpeas & Tahini

Feta & Rocket

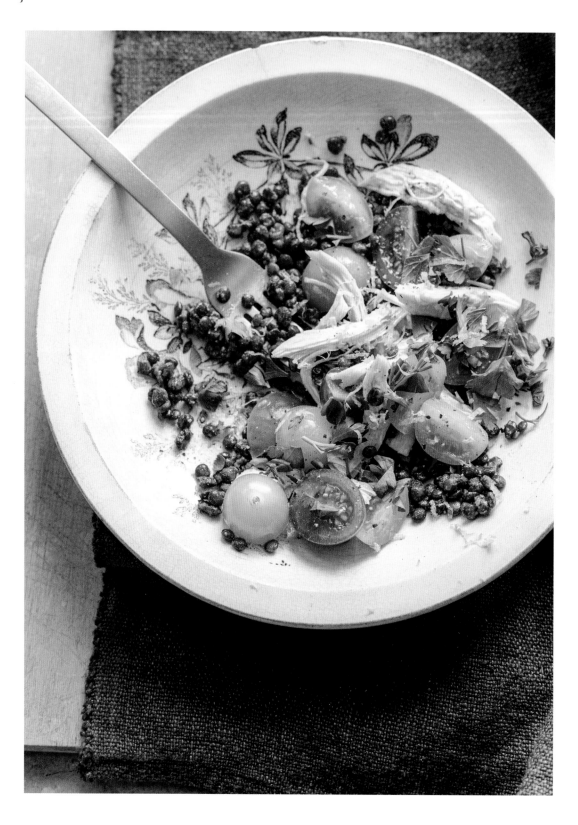

lentil & lemon chicken salad

{Serves 2}

The simplicity of this dish belies the flavour. It's such a staple in my life. Rocket, watercress and spinach are also good additions.

1 x 250g pouch of ready-cooked Puy lentils (I use Merchant Gourmet), or cook from scratch, according to the packet instructions*

zest and juice of 1 lemon

1 tablespoon tamari or soy sauce

1 tablespoon extra virgin olive oil

½ teaspoon garlic purée

1 portion of leftover roast chicken (approx. 150g)

1 large handful of fresh parsley, chopped

200g cherry tomatoes, roughly chopped

½ teaspoon sea salt

a pinch of freshly ground black pepper

Simply mix everything together well, and adjust the seasoning to taste.

This recipe is a great way of stretching out a small amount of leftover chicken to serve more people.

*
tip: Or use quinoa, bulgur wheat or cold, cooked pasta.

chicken, rocket & beetroot salad

{Serves 2}

Thanks to the beetroot, this is a beautiful pink salad using everyday fridge ingredients, pepped up with my go-to vinaigrette.

150g leftover roast chicken pieces

1 medium raw beetroot, peeled and grated (pre-cooked beetroot would also work – just chop rather than grate)

1 medium carrot, peeled and grated

8 cherry tomatoes, halved

2 handfuls of rocket (or any other salad leaves of your choice)

3 tablespoons pumpkin seeds

For the dressing

2 tablespoons extra virgin olive oil

3 tablespoons apple cider vinegar or white wine vinegar

1 teaspoon Dijon mustard

a pinch of sea salt

Mix the dressing ingredients together and divide between two 750ml jars or lunchboxes.

Layer the chicken and vegetables on top of the dressing, finishing with the salad leaves and pumpkin seeds.

Shake well before serving, so that the dressing coats the salad.

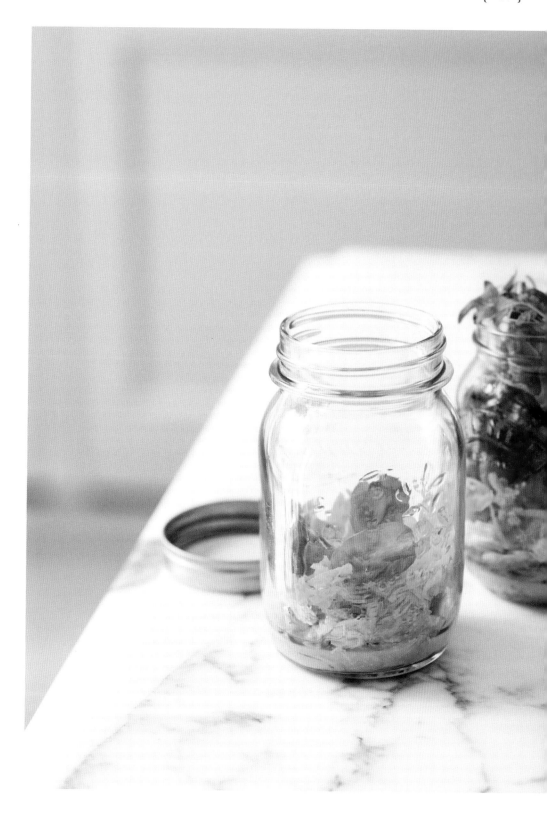

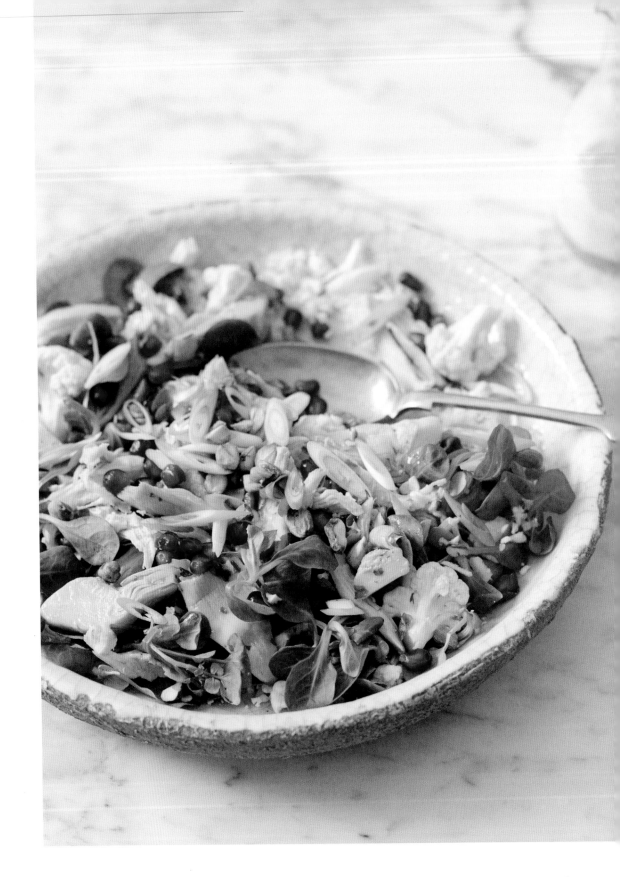

chicken, cauliflower & pistachio salad

{Serves 2}

I sometimes roast chicken specifically to make this salad. It is that good. Every mouthful is exciting.

150g leftover roast chicken pieces

30g pistachios, roughly chopped

1 bag of watercress (60g)

1 x 280g jar of artichoke hearts, drained of their oil

2 spring onions, sliced

2–3 large florets of cauliflower (approx. 150g), chopped

pomegranate seeds (optional)

For the dressing*

2 tablespoons plain yoghurt

1 tablespoon olive oil

6 fresh mint leaves, or 1 teaspoon dried mint

juice of ½ a lemon

a generous pinch of sea salt

Blend all the dressing ingredients together using a stick blender.

Mix all the salad ingredients together.

To pack your lunchbox, add half the dressing to the bottom of each box, then tumble the salad on top. Shake well before eating.

*
tip: If you're short on time, this is also lovely just drizzled with extra virgin olive oil, with a generous squeeze of lemon and a pinch of sea salt.

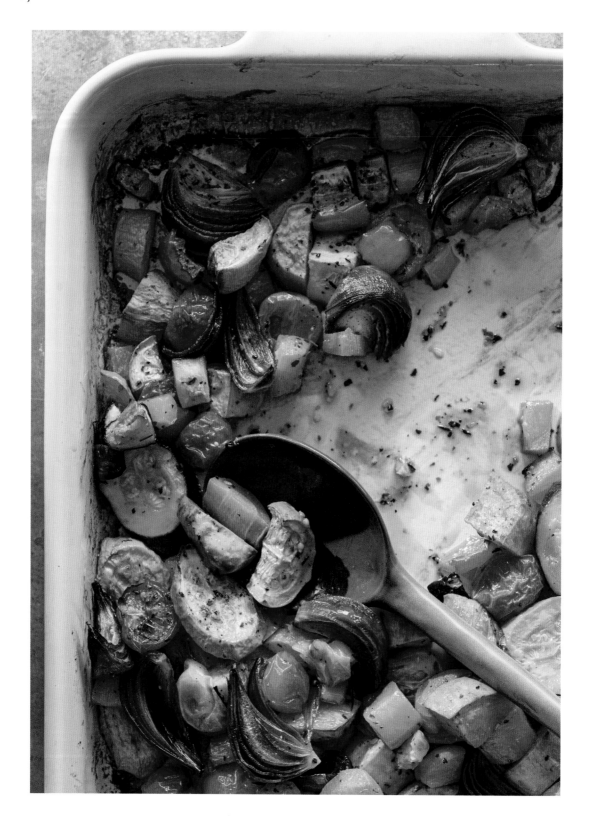

roasted vegetables (base recipe)

{Serves 4}

You can use any vegetables that you have to hand for this, so it is not a recipe that needs to be stuck to, more of an idea. The vegetables will keep in the fridge for 3 days.

2 **carrots**, washed and cut into 2cm bite-size cubes

2 **courgettes**, washed and cut into 2cm bite-size cubes

12 **cherry tomatoes**

1 **red pepper**, deseeded and cut into 2cm cubes

2 **small sweet potatoes**, peeled and cut into 2cm cubes

1 **red onion**, peeled and cut into thin wedges

2 tablespoons **olive oil**

sea salt and freshly ground black pepper

2 teaspoons **mixed dried herbs**

Heat the oven to 200°C/180°C fan.

Toss the vegetables with the olive oil, salt and pepper and the mixed dried herbs. Divide them between two non-stick baking trays and roast for 30 to 35 minutes, removing the trays from the oven to stir once or twice, until the vegetables are soft and starting to caramelize at the edges.

Eat straight away, or cool and store in the fridge for up to 3 days.

roasted vegetables, pesto, brown rice, pumpkin seeds & goat's cheese

{Serves 4}

This has long been a go-to lunch or supper for me, and my family all love it too. The rice can, of course, be swapped for quinoa, lentils, couscous or other, and the cheese can be swapped for feta, halloumi or Gorgonzola.
If you are plant based, omit the cheese and opt for vegan pesto, and add more nuts and seeds.

1 batch of Roasted Vegetables (see page 141)

4 tablespoons pumpkin seeds

2 x 250g pouches of cooked brown rice

150g pesto

125g soft goat's cheese

a few fresh basil leaves, to serve

If reheating the vegetables from fridge temperature, tip them into a large frying or sauté pan. Cover with a lid and cook over a medium heat for 5 to 10 minutes, stirring occasionally, until hot through. If the veg start to stick, add a splash of water.

Meanwhile, toast the pumpkin seeds in a small dry frying pan over a low-medium heat until they start to pop. Tip on to a plate and leave to cool.

Heat the rice according to the packet instructions.

Divide the rice between serving bowls. Stir the pesto into the vegetables and spoon on to the rice, then crumble over the goat's cheese and sprinkle with the toasted pumpkin seeds. Top with a few torn basil leaves.

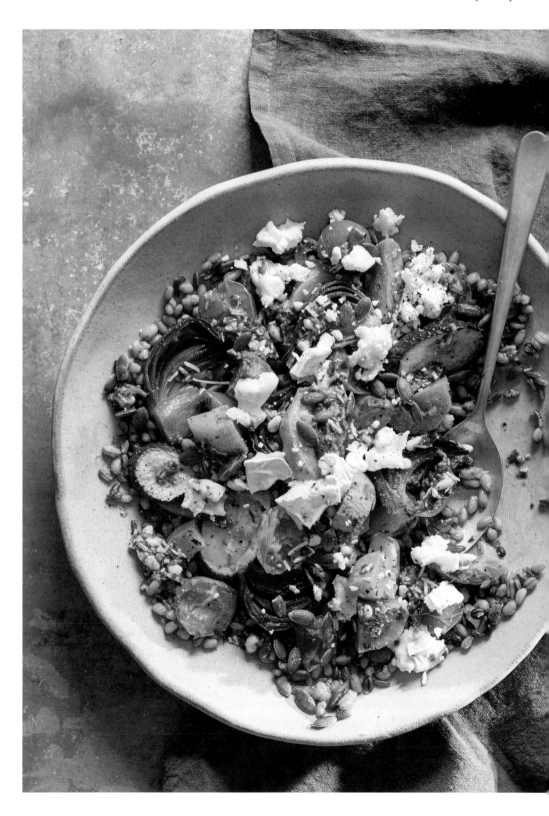

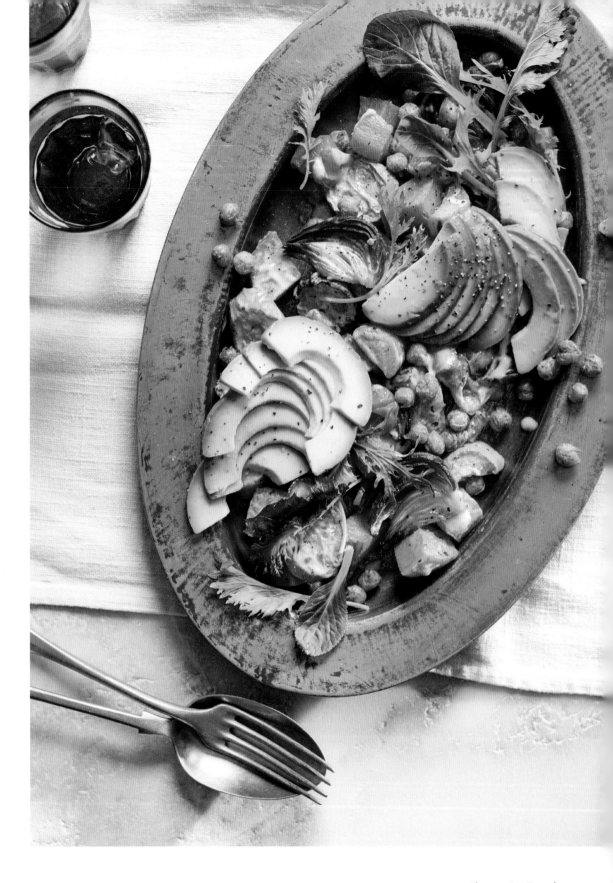

roasted vegetables, chickpeas & tahini

(vegan)

{Serves 4}

A rainbow of phytonutrients, vitamins and unrefined carbohydrates from the roasted vegetables; plant-based protein from the smoky chickpeas; and healthy fats from the creamy tahini and avocados. Balanced, simple and still very gratifying to eat.

2 x 400g tins of chickpeas, drained and rinsed

1 teaspoon smoked paprika

1 batch of Roasted Vegetables (see page 141)

1 x 60g bag of mixed salad leaves

2 avocados, peeled and sliced

For the dressing

3 tablespoons tahini

2 tablespoons white wine vinegar

1 teaspoon maple syrup or honey

2 tablespoons olive oil

sea salt and freshly ground black pepper

To make the dressing, whisk together the tahini, vinegar, maple syrup and 1 tablespoon of olive oil, and season with salt and pepper. The dressing will be very thick. Whisk in 2–3 tablespoons of hot water until it's a runny consistency.

Heat the remaining 1 tablespoon of oil in a large frying pan. Add the chickpeas and cook, stirring, on a high heat for 10 minutes, until starting to turn golden. Add the smoked paprika and some salt and pepper, and stir for another minute to coat the chickpeas. Tip the chickpeas on to a plate.

If reheating the roasted vegetables from fridge temperature, tip them into the frying pan. Cook, covered, on a medium heat for 5 to 10 minutes, stirring occasionally, until hot through. Add a splash of water if needed. Remove from the heat and stir in 2 tablespoons of the dressing.

Spoon the vegetables into bowls and top with the crispy chickpeas. Drizzle with the remaining dressing and serve with salad leaves and avocado slices.

roasted vegetable, feta & rocket salad

{Serves 4}
great to make ahead
for taking to work

Salads can be among the very best food we can eat, when made with imagination and care. Many people tell me they find salads boring or can't move past lettuce, cucumber and tomato. But there are endless potential flavour combinations and peppy ingredients to try. This is a perennial, speedy favourite of mine which is also a great option to make ahead and take to work.

1 batch of Roasted Vegetables (see page 141)

1 tablespoon sunflower seeds

1 bag of rocket or mixed salad leaves

100g feta, crumbled

extra virgin olive oil

balsamic vinegar

sea salt and freshly ground black pepper

Tumble the roasted vegetables and seeds into a bowl with a big handful of rocket or salad leaves, and a little crumbled feta.

Drizzle with olive oil and a little balsamic, and season with salt and pepper.

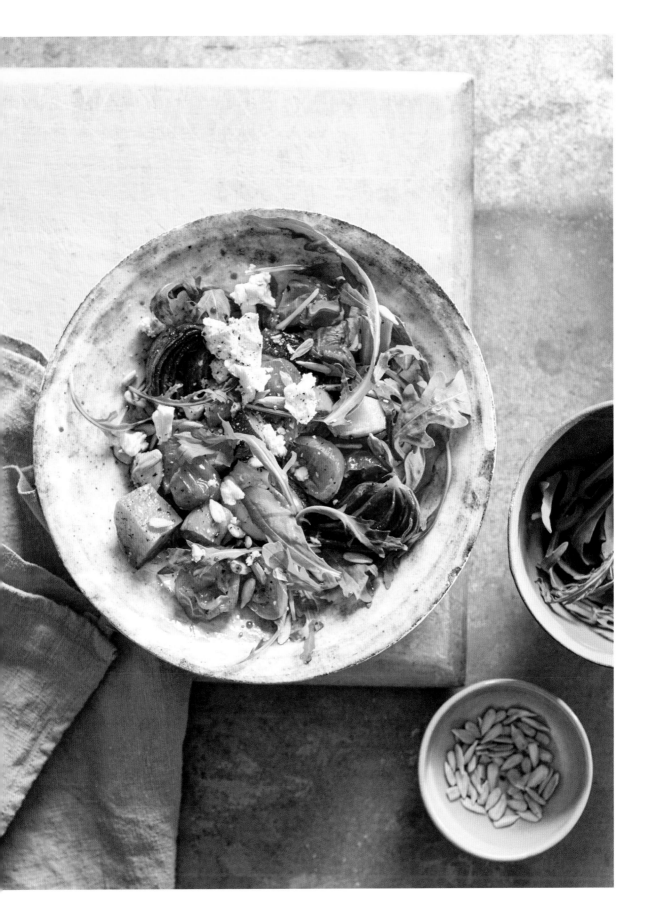

spinach & beetroot falafel

{Makes 10}

My daughter loves falafels, so I make them alot. I make a bigger batch than I need and freeze half for another occasion. For grown-ups, I'll put them into a wrap with yoghurt, sliced red onion, tomato, beetroot, cucumber and a big handful of rocket.

1 x 400g tin of chickpeas, drained and rinsed

2 handfuls of spinach

1 teaspoon ground cumin

2 cloves of garlic, peeled and crushed

1 cooked beetroot

2 tablespoons chopped fresh parsley

1 teaspoon sea salt

1 teaspoon baking powder

1 tablespoon lemon juice

4–5 tablespoons wholemeal flour or Doves Farm Gluten Free

3 tablespoons olive oil, to fry

Put everything apart from the flour and oil into a food processor and blitz until the mixture is coming together but still has a bit of texture. Stir in the flour 1 tablespoon at a time until the mixture is firm enough to shape into balls.

Damp your hands to shape into golfball-size patties, flattening them a little with your hand. Heat the oil in a frying pan and fry the patties in batches until golden on both sides. This should take 2 minutes or so.

Can be eaten hot or cold – perfect with roasted vegetables and houmous.

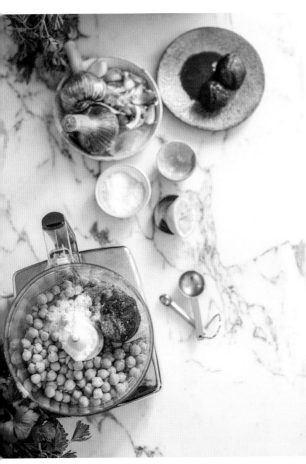

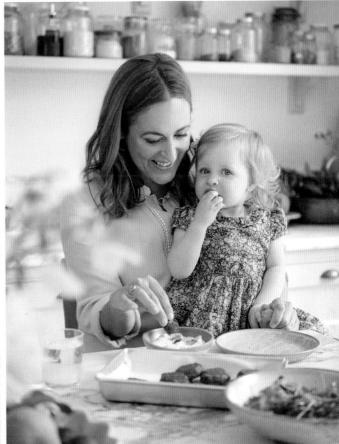

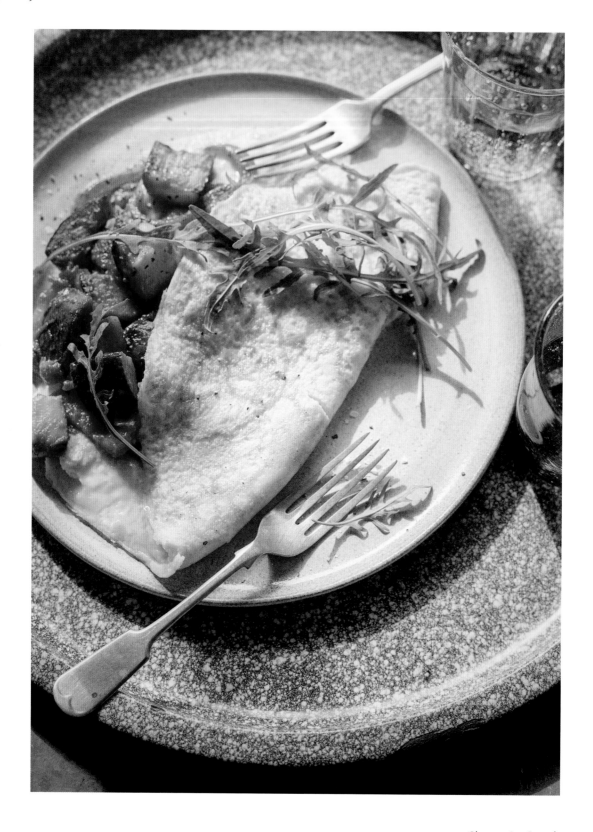

ratatouille omelette

{Serves 2}

There couldn't be a simpler meal than an omelette and I frequently turn to it. Here I have paired it with some ratatouille, which is something I also often make, but it works just as well with some leftover cooked vegetables, sliced greens, grated cheese and spring onion or a handful of fresh herbs.

For the ratatouille

olive oil

1 courgette, cut into 2cm chunks

1 aubergine, cut into 2cm chunks

1 red pepper, cut into 3cm chunks

1 red onion, peeled and cut into thin wedges

½ teaspoon mixed dried herbs

a pinch of chilli flakes (optional)

sea salt and freshly ground black pepper

1 x 400g tin of chopped tomatoes

For the omelette

4 large eggs

olive oil

To serve

a handful of rocket

For the ratatouille
Heat some olive oil in a large frying pan. Tip in the courgettes, aubergines, red peppers and red onions along with the herbs, chilli flakes, if using, and seasoning, and fry until just soft.

Stir in the chopped tomatoes with a small splash of water and cook for another 10 to 15 minutes, until the sauce has reduced slightly.

For the omelette
Whisk the eggs in a bowl. Heat a small flat non-stick pan over a medium-high heat. Add a splash of oil and, once hot, tip in the eggs. As they cook, use the corner of a fish slice to draw the cooked egg into the middle so that the raw egg runs out to the sides of the pan. Once nearly cooked, fold the omelette in half and slide on to a serving plate. Cut in half, and serve with a large spoonful of warm ratatouille and a handful of rocket leaves.

mushroom & sage chicken liver pâté

{Serves 4 to 6}

After having my daughter, I found myself craving pâté (something I rarely eat). I think it was my body's way of helping replenish lost nutrients as liver is particularly high in iron and vitamin B12.

3 cloves of garlic, peeled and crushed

2 red onions, peeled and diced

2–3 tablespoons olive oil

300g chestnut mushrooms, roughly chopped

1 level teaspoon sea salt

5–6 fresh sage leaves (optional), chopped, plus extra for garnish

300g organic chicken livers, roughly chopped*

In a heavy-bottomed pan or casserole, sauté the garlic and onions in the olive oil over a low-medium heat, until they are soft – about 5 minutes. Add the chopped mushrooms, and cook over a medium heat for 5 minutes until these too have softened and started to release their water.

Finally, add the salt, chopped sage and chicken livers. Stir the mix well. Cover with a lid, and gently cook for around 15 minutes, stirring occasionally, until the livers are thoroughly cooked through and no longer pink. Remove the lid, and allow the mixture to cool until just warm.

Use a slotted spoon to transfer the mix into a blender (you may need to add some of the cooking juices to achieve the right consistency), and blend for 2 to 3 minutes, or until completely smooth.

Cool and leave in the fridge to thicken. Consume within 2 to 3 days, or freeze. Serve garnished with sage leaves.

*
tip: With livers, I really try to buy only organic, so I am opportunistic when I come across them – they freeze well from fresh – for use another day.

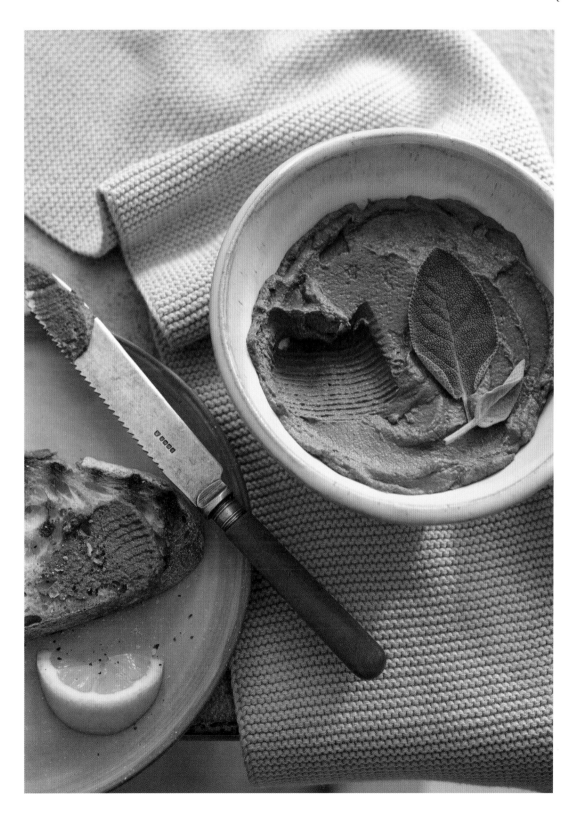

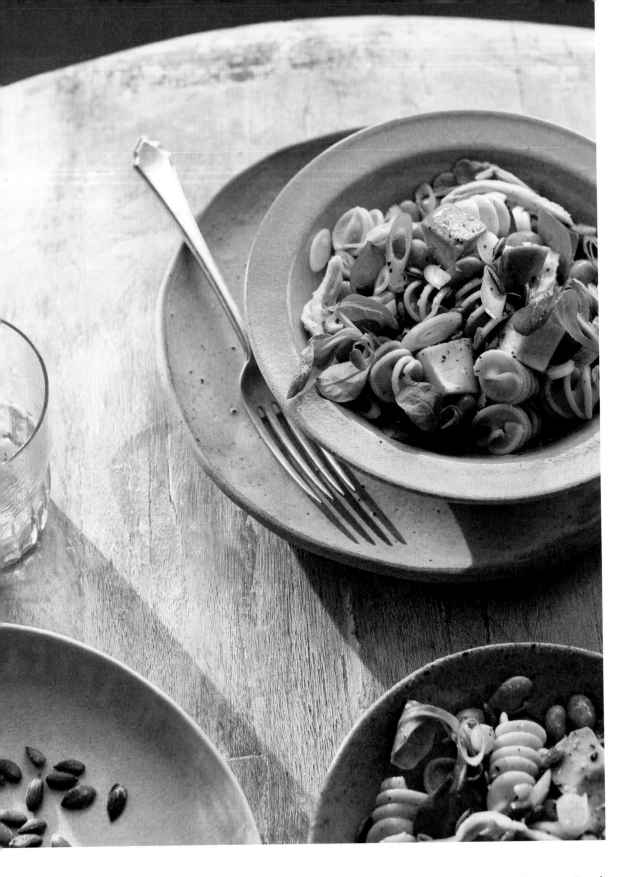

green chopped chicken & chickpea pasta salad with miso sesame dressing

{Serves 4}

Variety is key in our diet. So instead of always using the same pasta, I like to use different ones. Legume pastas such as chickpea, lentil and pea are now widely available in big supermarkets. They are naturally gluten-free and are generally higher in protein as well as offering a different profile of nutrients to wheat pasta. By all means stick to whichever pasta you prefer, but I do love the slightly nuttier taste of the chickpea pasta in this salad. Take care not to overcook legume pastas, as they can go quite soggy. If you can't find frozen soya beans for this recipe, you can substitute baby broad beans or peas instead.

200g chickpea pasta

150g frozen soya beans (edamame beans)

150g cooked chicken, shredded

½ an avocado, peeled and cut into cubes

15g toasted pumpkin seeds

2 handfuls of lamb's lettuce

1 spring onion, sliced

For the dressing*

1 teaspoon miso paste

1 tablespoon light olive oil

3 tablespoons rice vinegar

1 teaspoon honey

1 teaspoon tamari/soy or coconut amino sauce

1 teaspoon sesame seeds

1 teaspoon sesame oil

sea salt and freshly ground black pepper

Put the chickpea pasta on to cook according to the packet instructions. Add the frozen soya beans for the last 2 minutes of the cooking time. Drain, then run under cold water.

For the dressing, simply blend all the ingredients together either in a bowl with a whisk, or in a blender.

Toss everything together in a bowl with the dressing, and serve.

*
tip: It's worth making double quantities of the dressing to elevate future meals with a flavourful punch. Keep it in a jar in the fridge for up to a week.

vegetable & feta fritters

{Makes 8}

You can use up any sad-looking leftover vegetables from the fridge to make these fritters. I have used a couple of courgettes and a carrot here, but a whole plethora of vegetables would work – chopped leaves, grated beetroot, finely diced peppers, parsnips or squash – be creative.

100g feta, crumbled

2 medium courgettes, grated and squeezed well to remove excess water

1 medium carrot, peeled, grated and squeezed well in a j-cloth/muslin to remove excess water

1½ teaspoons ground coriander

½ teaspoon sea salt

4 tablespoons ground almonds

1 egg

zest of ½ a lemon

olive oil

Mix together all the ingredients, apart from the oil, in a large mixing bowl, until well combined. Then, using wet hands, roughly shape into 8 patties.

Heat some olive oil in a large heavy-based frying pan, and fry in batches for a few minutes on each side, or until golden.

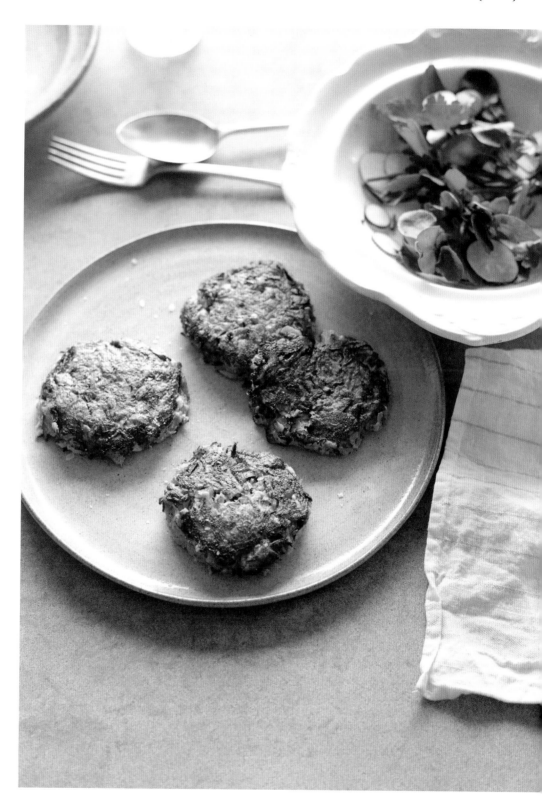

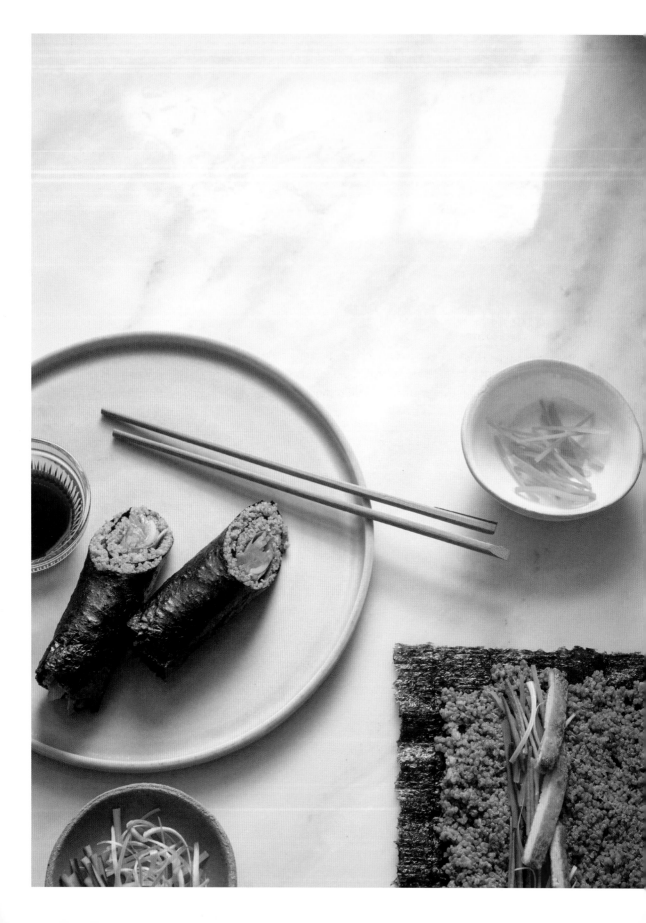

nori wraps
(vegan)

{Serves 4}

Nori is a type of seaweed that you can usually find in the 'World Foods' section of the supermarket, and is most often used to make sushi. It provides us with a source of iodine – a key mineral that those on a plant-based diet, or who can't consume dairy, may be at risk of being low in. These wraps are quite hands-on to make, so are ideal for getting children involved.

1 medium, ripe avocado

2 tablespoons apple cider vinegar

a pinch of sea salt

250g cooked quinoa
(I usually just use a pre-cooked packet)

8 sheets of nori seaweed

Cut the avocado in half, remove the flesh and mash it with the back of a fork in a small bowl, along with the vinegar and a pinch of salt. Add the cooked quinoa, and mix thoroughly. The mashed avocado should start to bind the quinoa together a little.

Take one sheet of nori and spread a couple of tablespoons of the quinoa mixture out at one end of the sheet. Pile your chosen fillings on top and roll up tightly. You can brush a little water on the join to help it stick together.

Slice each wrap in half at an angle. Repeat with the remaining sheets of nori and the rest of the filling.

Filling suggestions
Use a selection of the following (what you have in the fridge, or enjoy eating):

~ thin carrot batons

~ thin cucumber batons

~ extra slices of avocado

~ fine slices of spring onion

~ rocket or spinach

~ coriander

~ tuna, smoked mackerel or smoked salmon

~ fried or grilled tofu strips

~ quartered hard-boiled eggs

~ houmous

~ seed sprouts

DINNER
3}

fishcakes

Having some fish in the freezer is a useful back-up when the fridge is empty and we've got hungry mouths to feed. However, frozen fish can often be dry and lacklustre compared to fresh, which can understandably put people off this handy staple. These fishcakes are a brilliant solution, with the added bonus of avoiding having to peel and boil potatoes, as the chickpeas provide the carbohydrate and bulk.

{Serves 4}

1 x 400g tin of chickpeas, drained and rinsed

a handful of fresh parsley (or baby leaf spinach)

1 spring onion, sliced

zest and juice of ½ a lemon

2–3 skinless, frozen fish fillets, ideally thawed (2 medium, or 3 if they are small)

1 small egg, beaten

sea salt and freshly ground black pepper

light olive oil

Pulse the chickpeas, parsley, spring onion, lemon zest and juice in a food processor a few times. Don't over-mix, or you'll end up with houmous.

Add the fish fillets and pulse two or three more times – just enough to break the fish up and mix it through. Pour the mixture into a mixing bowl and stir in the beaten egg. This will help to bind the mixture. Season with salt and pepper.

Form the mixture into 8 small patties using damp hands (or spoons).

Heat a large non-stick frying pan over a medium heat and add a generous amount of light olive oil. Fry the patties in batches for 6 minutes each side, or until golden brown. Don't be tempted to turn them until they have really crisped up on the bottom, as they have a tendency to fall apart.

tip: Leave the mixture to set in the fridge for 10 to 15 minutes if you have time. This will make the patties easier to shape. You can also use pre-cooked fish in this recipe, such as hot smoked trout, poached salmon or white fish. The best way to poach salmon is to put it into cold water, bring to the boil, simmer for 2 minutes, then take off the heat and allow the salmon to sit in the water for a few minutes to finish cooking.

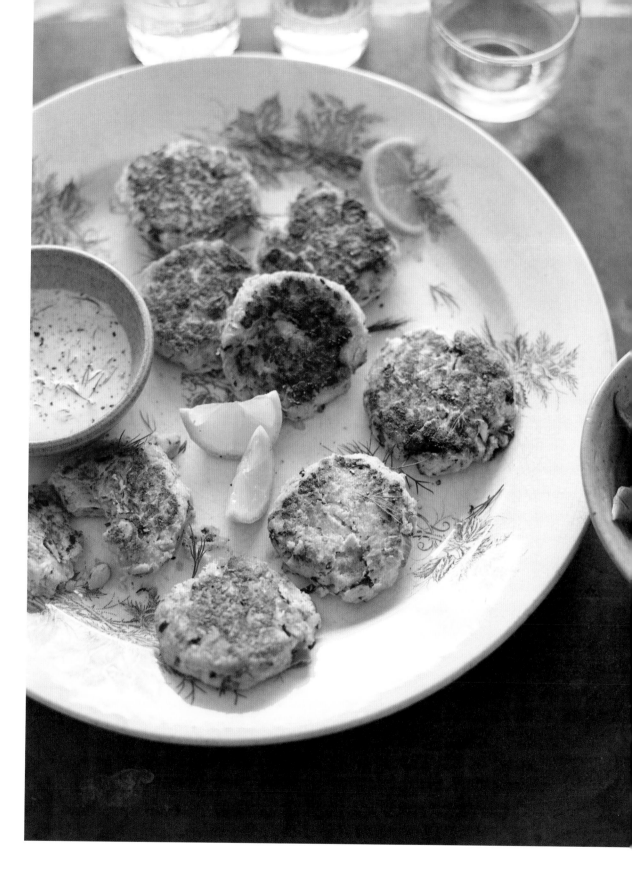

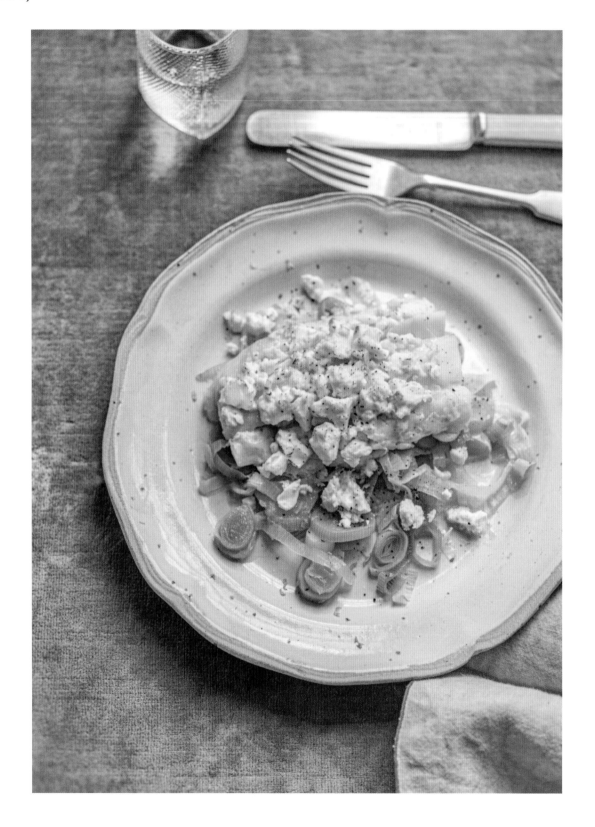

cod, feta & leek bake

The very simplest of suppers, with just three main ingredients, but don't dismiss it as bland, as it is in fact silky on the tongue and creamy, not heavy. Cooking length will vary depending on how thick the fish fillet is (cod or hake work really well here, but so would salmon). If in doubt, pull the dish out of the oven a couple of minutes early, and take a look at the centre of the fillet with a knife. If it is opaque all the way through, it's done. If not, put it back in and check again after another 2 to 3 minutes. This is lovely as it is, but some peas, steamed greens and/or new potatoes would make it more filling if needed.

{Serves 2}

2 large leeks, trimmed and sliced

2 fish fillets, skinless (cod works particularly well), fresh or frozen

olive oil

75g feta

zest of ½ a lemon

Preheat the oven to 200°C/180°C fan.

Steam the leeks for 5 minutes, or until softened. Once cooked, spread them over the bottom of a small baking dish.

Place the fish on top of the leeks and drizzle generously with olive oil. Crumble the feta, using your fingers, over the top of the fish.

Bake for 25 minutes (from frozen) or 8 to 12 minutes (from thawed).

Serve immediately, sprinkled with lemon zest.

fish & pesto parcels

{Serves 2}

I make fresh pesto throughout the summer and freeze it in small portions or ice cube trays to use at other times of year. It's a great way to add a quick pop of flavour and some nutrients, especially if you pack in lots of greens. You can of course buy really delicious pesto if you don't make your own. With only three ingredients, this recipe is quick and easy and something I make again and again. As always, vegetables are king so serve this with a handful of lettuce leaves or some steamed or sautéed greens.

2 fish fillets of choice, skinless, fresh or frozen

2 heaped teaspoons good-quality pesto (look for one made with olive oil rather than sunflower oil)

1 large tomato, sliced

3 new potatoes and a handful of greens per person, to serve

Preheat the oven to 200°C/180°C fan.

Arrange each fillet on a large square of baking parchment. Top with pesto (1 teaspoon over each), followed by a few slices of tomato.

Fold the top and sides of each piece of parchment together, to make two sealed parcels. Place them on a baking tray. Bake for 25 to 30 minutes (from frozen) or 10 to 15 minutes (fresh), depending on the size of the fillets.

While the fish is in the oven, boil the new potatoes for 8 to 10 minutes, steaming the greens at the same time (I like to use spinach). Crush the potatoes with a little olive oil, salt and pepper.

Serve the fish hot, with the potatoes and greens.

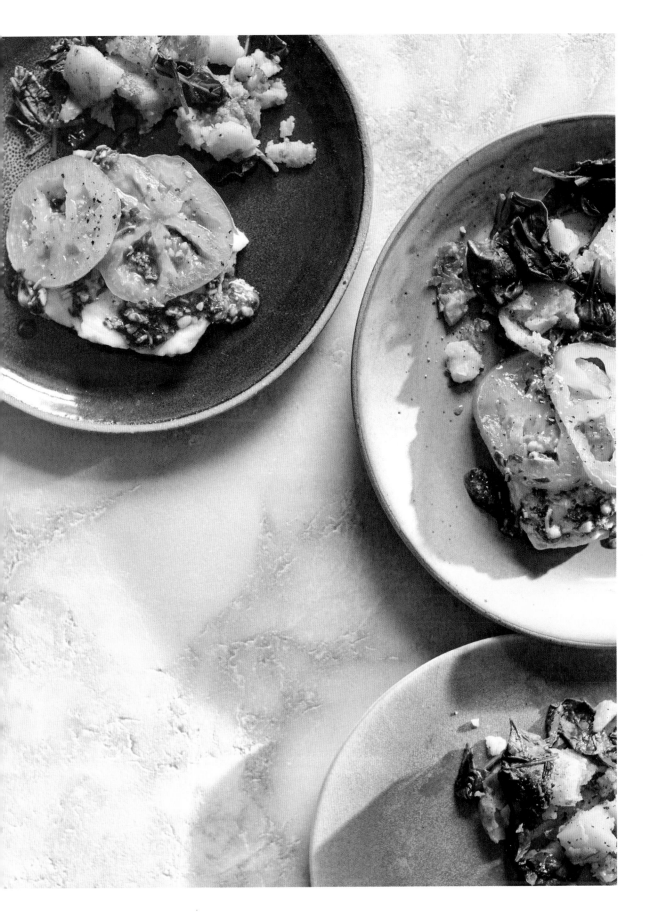

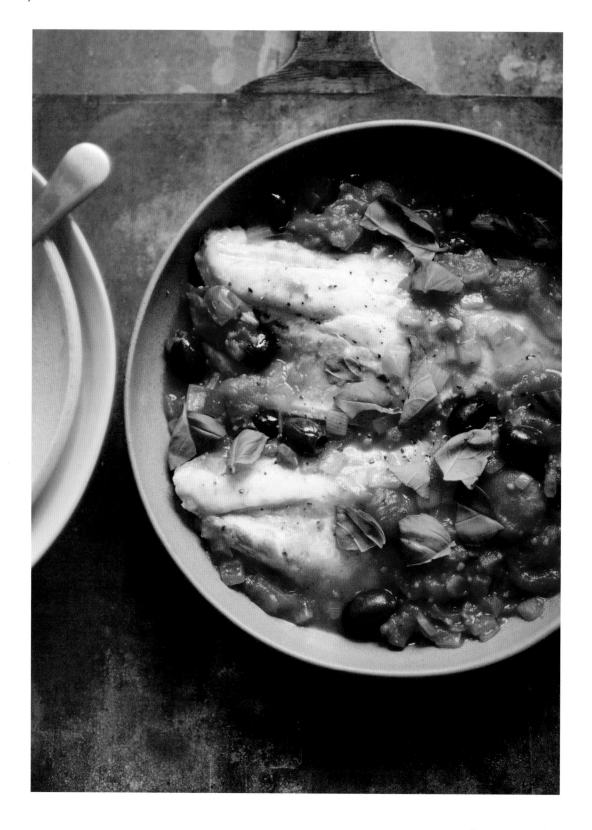

fish provençale

{Serves 4}

Provençale sauce is a really versatile and fragrant sauce that can be used to liven up the most basic of meals from pasta, jacket potatoes, chicken or fish, as here. If you feel you need something more filling, add some wholegrain rice or pasta or a serving of courgetti.

1 **onion**, peeled and diced

1 **clove of garlic**, peeled and crushed

olive oil

1 x 400g tin of **cherry tomatoes**

70g **pitted black olives**

4 **fish fillets**, frozen or fresh

fresh basil, to finish

This works best in a shallow frying pan with a lid, although a large cast-iron casserole with a lid can also be used.

Sauté the onion and garlic together in a little olive oil for 8 to 10 minutes, until soft. Add the cherry tomatoes and black olives and bring to a very gentle simmer.

Top with the fish fillets and cover with the lid. Poach for 10 to 20 minutes (depending on the size of the fish and if it is fresh or frozen. It is done when opaque all the way through and flakes easily).

Serve hot, sprinkled with torn basil leaves.

summer
salmon
in a bag

{Serves 2}

Because the baking parchment traps in steam during cooking, the fish stays deliciously moist. To check if it is cooked through, unfold the packet and take a peek. It should be opaque almost the whole way through. If the fish needs a few more minutes, tightly rewrap the packet before giving it another couple of minutes, so you don't lose any moisture in the oven.

zest and juice of 1 lemon

sea salt and freshly ground black pepper

1 courgette (approx. 300g), spiralized or sliced into rounds

8 cherry tomatoes, halved

a small handful of spinach leaves (50g)

1 x 400g tin of butter beans, drained and rinsed

2 x 200g salmon fillets

a few sprigs of fresh herbs

4 tablespoons olive oil

mixed green salad leaves, to serve

Preheat the oven to 220°C/200°C fan. Cut an 80cm length of baking parchment and lay half of it on a flat baking tray, with the other half hanging over the edge.

In a medium bowl, whisk together half the lemon juice, 1 teaspoon of sea salt and a few grinds of pepper. Add the courgettes, cherry tomatoes, spinach and drained butter beans. Toss to combine.

Use a slotted spoon to put the veg and bean mixture in the centre of the prepared baking tray. Keep back any liquid left in the bowl.

Dip the salmon fillets into the reserved liquid, then place them on top of the pile of vegetables. Season with pepper and lay the herbs on top (if you have them).

Fold the baking parchment over, pleating the edges to seal. Bake for 15 minutes.

Once cooked, take out of the oven and leave on the tray, covered, for 5 more minutes. The last bit of steam will finish the cooking process.

Open the parcel and add the olive oil, the rest of the lemon juice, and a little lemon zest.

Serve with the salad leaves.

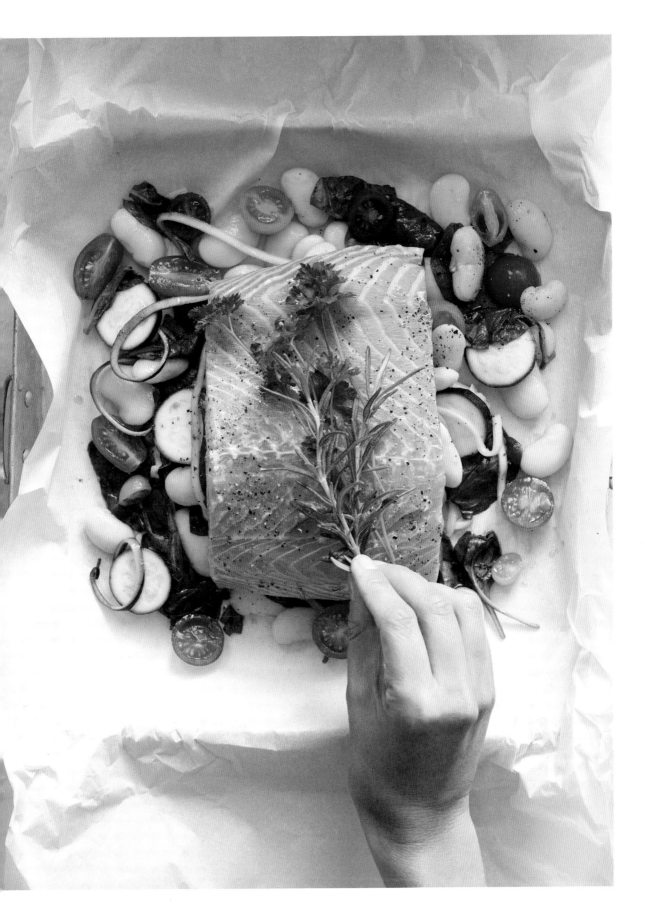

spicy fish with a herby broccoli mash

I have used cod here, but any white fish or salmon would work. The broccoli makes a lovely mashed potato substitute, but if you are ravenous, add a few steamed potatoes too.

{Serves 1}

180g cod fillet, skinless

1 tablespoon harissa paste

½ a lemon, sliced

6–8 cherry tomatoes

a pinch of sea salt flakes

200g broccoli (1 small head), cut into small florets

3 tablespoons olive oil

a few leaves of fresh basil and coriander

½ teaspoon sea salt

freshly ground black pepper

juice of ½ a lemon

Preheat the oven to 200°C/180°C fan.

Coat the fish with the harissa and place it on a baking tray. Lay the lemon slices on top, and toss the cherry tomatoes around the fish. Sprinkle over a pinch of sea salt flakes and bake for 15 minutes.

Meanwhile, steam the broccoli florets for 5 to 7 minutes, until tender but still bright green.

Put the cooked broccoli into a blender with the olive oil, herbs, salt and pepper and pulse into a chunky mash.

Serve with a squeeze of lemon juice.

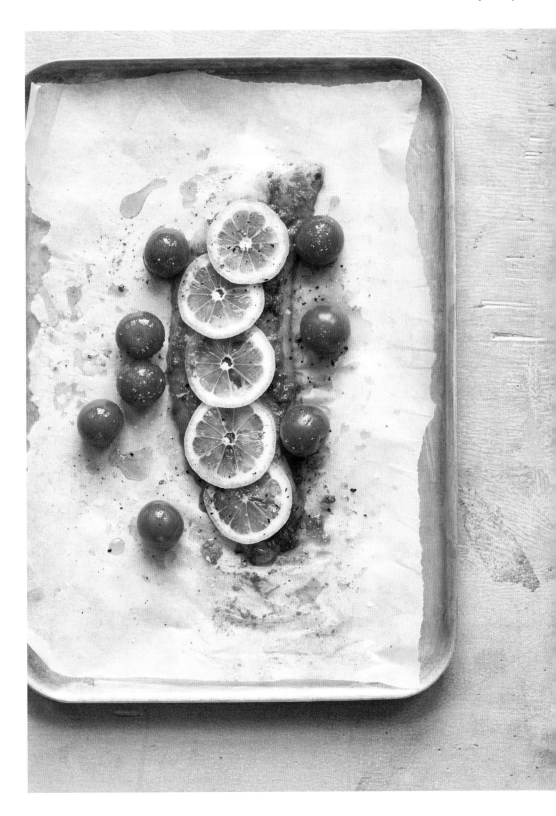

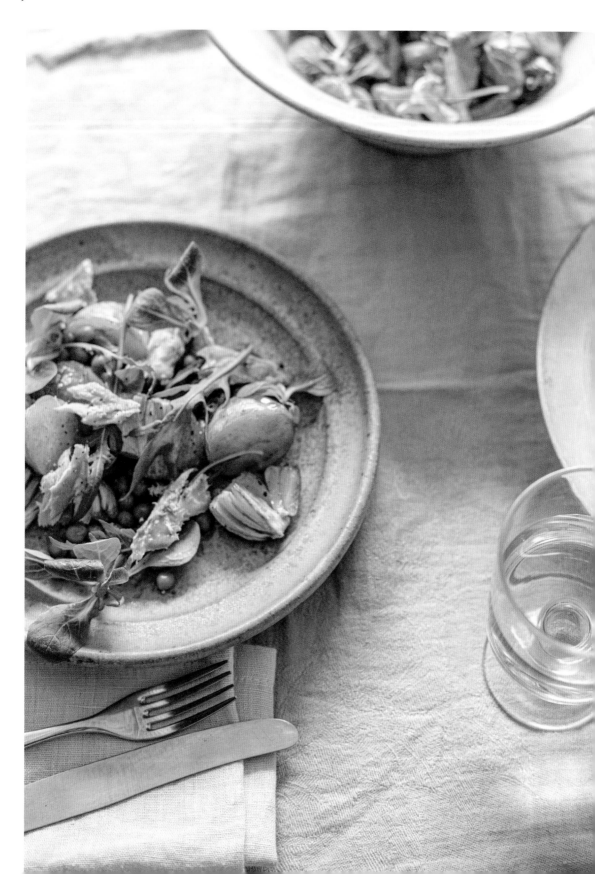

warm lemony mackerel & new potato salad

{Serves 2}

This is the kind of meal this book was created for. Deliciously straightforward everyday food. The mackerel could be substituted for flaked poached or smoked salmon or trout. It's just as delicious cold.

200g new potatoes, halved (leave the skins on)

1 large bulb of fennel, roughly chopped

olive oil

150g frozen peas (or frozen broad beans)

2–3 fillets of smoked mackerel

2 handfuls of salad leaves of your choice (I like watercress, rocket or spinach)

juice of ½ a lemon

Preheat the oven to 200°C /180°C fan.

Toss the new potatoes and fennel into a roasting tin, and drizzle with a little olive oil. Roast for 35 to 40 minutes, until cooked through and golden at the edges. Add the peas for the final few minutes of cooking, to heat them through.

Allow to cool slightly, then transfer to a serving bowl.

Tear the mackerel fillets into bite-size pieces, and mix through the vegetables. Add the salad leaves and a generous squeeze of lemon juice to taste.

Serve warm.

harissa prawn skewers with herbed broccoli rice

{Serves 2}

Harissa paste is the first thing I reach for when I need to add good flavour and quickly. There are many brands, some of which are spicier than others and some that have a lot more ingredients than others, so read the labels when choosing. I was surprised and delighted when Willow first tried it and loved it. This is a gem of a recipe that exudes flavour but isn't heavy. It's an absolute treat to make and eat.

1 head of broccoli

20 raw king prawns

12 cherry tomatoes

1 tablespoon harissa paste

1 tablespoon coconut or olive oil

1 teaspoon sea salt

a grind of black pepper

juice of ½ a lemon

1 tablespoon chopped fresh basil

1 tablespoon chopped fresh mint

lime wedges, to serve

To make the broccoli rice, chop the broccoli into florets and pulse in a food processor until the texture resembles rice.

Turn the grill to high. Put the prawns and tomatoes into a bowl and add the harissa and oil. Season with the sea salt and black pepper.

Thread the prawns and tomatoes on to four skewers. (Note: if using wooden ones, soak them in water for at least 15 minutes before using, to prevent them from burning under the grill.) Grill for 4 to 6 minutes, until the prawns are pink, turning halfway through.

Meanwhile, heat a frying pan. Add the broccoli rice with 1 tablespoon of water and cook for 3 minutes, stirring all the time. Add the lemon juice and season with salt and pepper, then take off the heat and stir in the chopped herbs.

Serve the skewers hot from the grill, with the broccoli rice and wedges of lime.

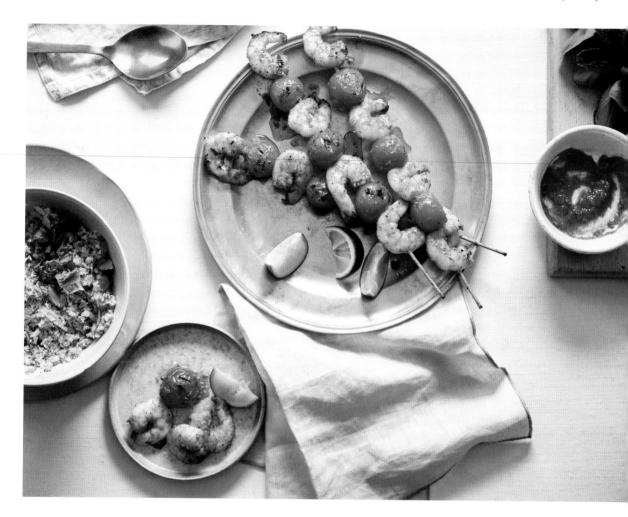

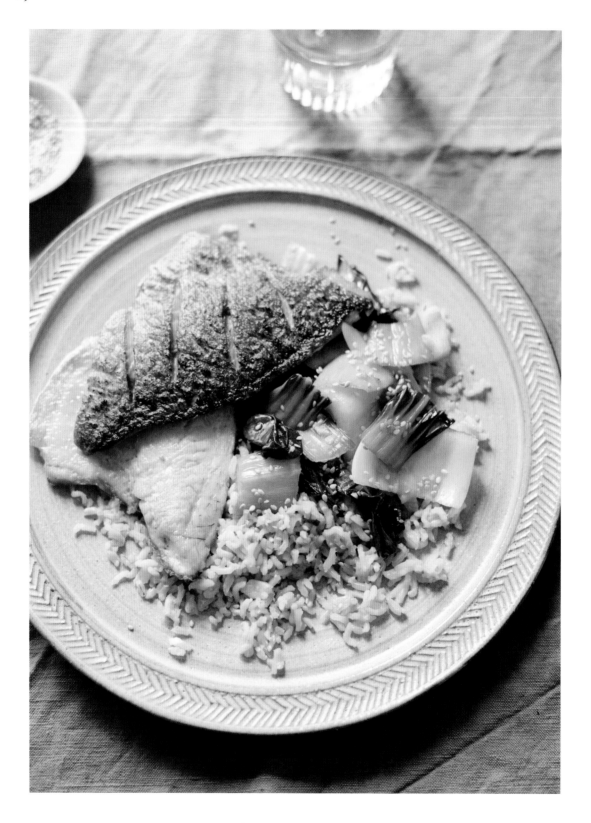

pan-fried sea bream with pak choi & tamari sauce

{Serves 1}

You can use any white fish for this recipe or salmon or trout. You may need to adjust the cooking times slightly according to the thickness of the fillets you choose. This dish can be eaten just as it is or, if you feel like something more substantial, add brown basmati rice.

50g brown basmati rice, rinsed until the water runs clear, and drained (optional)

1 teaspoon white sesame seeds

2 fillets of sea bream (approx. 125g)

1 tablespoon extra virgin olive oil

1 teaspoon finely diced fresh ginger

150–200g pak choi (2 heads), washed and chopped

1 tablespoon tamari

juice of ½ a lime

2 teaspoons maple syrup

2 teaspoons fish sauce

If you are using the rice, cook it according to the packet instructions and put to one side – it will keep its heat while you get on with cooking the fish and greens.

Heat a large, lidded non-stick frying pan. Once hot, add the white sesame seeds. Keep shaking the pan until you hear the seeds pop and see them get some colour. Put the toasted seeds aside in a bowl.

Slash the skin side of the sea bream fillets, using a sharp knife. Put some olive oil into the frying pan, then add the fish, skin side down. Reduce the heat to low and fry for 5 minutes on the skin side only, until golden brown and completely cooked through. Turn them over to 'kiss' the pan with the flesh side down for a quick minute, then remove and keep warm.

Using the same pan, add the diced ginger and the pak choi, giving a quick stir to coat and incorporate the oil and ginger, then cover the pan. The leftover water on the leaves (from being washed) will help steam the greens – 2 to 3 minutes should be enough.

Meanwhile mix together the tamari, lime juice, maple syrup, fish sauce and sesame seeds in a bowl. Pour into the pan with the greens and turn off the heat.

Serve the fish and pak choi with the rice (if using) and any leftover juices from the pan.

tip: A little tip for peeling ginger is just to scrape the skin with a teaspoon – it peels off very easily – then freeze any left over, which make it very easy to grate.

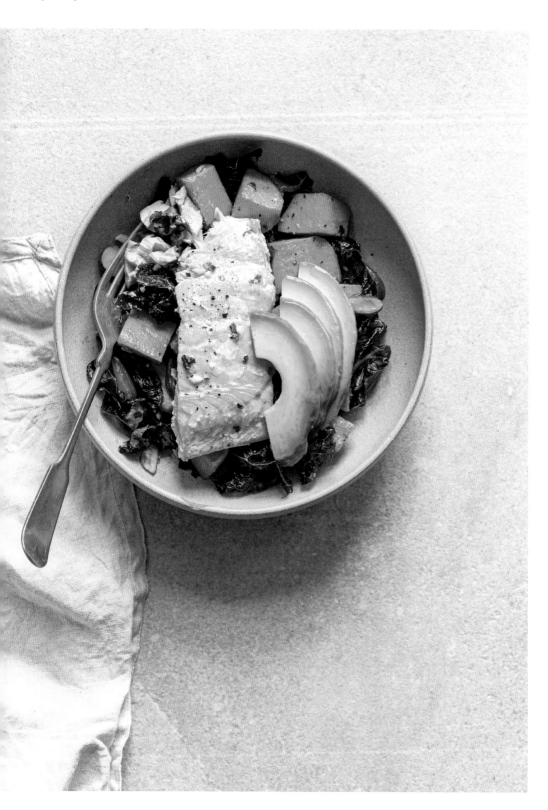

roasted salmon with sweet potato & kale

A balanced, nutritious meal made from readily available ingredients, all roasted on one tray. Simple.

{Serves 2}

1 sweet potato (approx. 200g), peeled and cut into cubes

2 wild salmon fillets

2 handfuls of kale leaves, ribs removed and chopped

30g slivered almonds

½ an avocado, sliced

For the dressing

2 tablespoons olive oil

2 tablespoons tamari (or soy or coconut amino sauce)

juice of ½ a lemon

⅛ teaspoon chilli flakes

sea salt and freshly ground black pepper

Preheat the oven to 200°C/180°C fan.

Mix together the olive oil, tamari, lemon juice, chilli flakes, salt and pepper to make the dressing.

Lay the sweet potato cubes on a baking tray and drizzle with a third of the dressing. Roast for 10 minutes. Add the salmon (skin side down), kale and almonds to the tray and pour over a little more of the dressing, keeping some back. Roast for another 10 minutes, being careful that the kale and nuts don't burn and turn bitter. The sweet potato needs to be soft on the inside and golden on the outside and the salmon needs to be cooked through (or to your liking).

Remove the salmon fillets from the tray. Toss all the vegetables together and put into bowls, then add the avocado and place the salmon on top. Serve with the rest of the dressing drizzled over.

za'atar chicken, aubergine & squash traybake

{Serves 6}

Traybakes are among the simplest dishes to make. Bung everything into one tray – vegetables, meat or fish and flavours – and roast it all together in the oven. No fuss, great flavours and minimal washing-up. This particular combination is a personal favourite of mine. Za'atar is a Middle Eastern spice blend. You can find it in most big supermarkets now, but if it's difficult to get hold of, just substitute dried oregano and ground cumin instead.

12 chicken thigh fillets
(skin removed)

1 butternut squash, peeled
and diced into rough cubes

2 medium aubergines,
diced into rough cubes

4 tablespoons olive oil

4 tablespoons za'atar
(or 1 teaspoon dried
oregano + 2 teaspoons
ground cumin)

2 onions, peeled and
cut into quarters

3 cloves of garlic, peeled
and crushed

sea salt and freshly
ground black pepper

Preheat the oven to 200°C/180°C fan.

In a large mixing bowl, drizzle the chicken thigh fillets, butternut squash and aubergines with the olive oil, then scatter over the za'atar. Mix well to coat each piece with the flavour and oil. Tip on to a large roasting tray (you may need to use two) and add the onion quarters and the garlic. Season with salt and pepper.

Roast for around 30 to 40 minutes, or until the vegetables are soft and the chicken is cooked all the way through – with no hint of pink in the middle.

Serve simply with a rocket salad or some steamed seasonal greens on the side. Or if you would like to make it a little bit more special, serve topped with a pile of chopped coriander and some pomegranate seeds, perhaps with some steamed new potatoes and a feta-dotted herby salad too.

tip: This makes a great leftover dish to take to work for lunch the next day. Just stir through lots of salad leaves and (if you are feeling fancy) a sprinkling of pomegranate seeds.

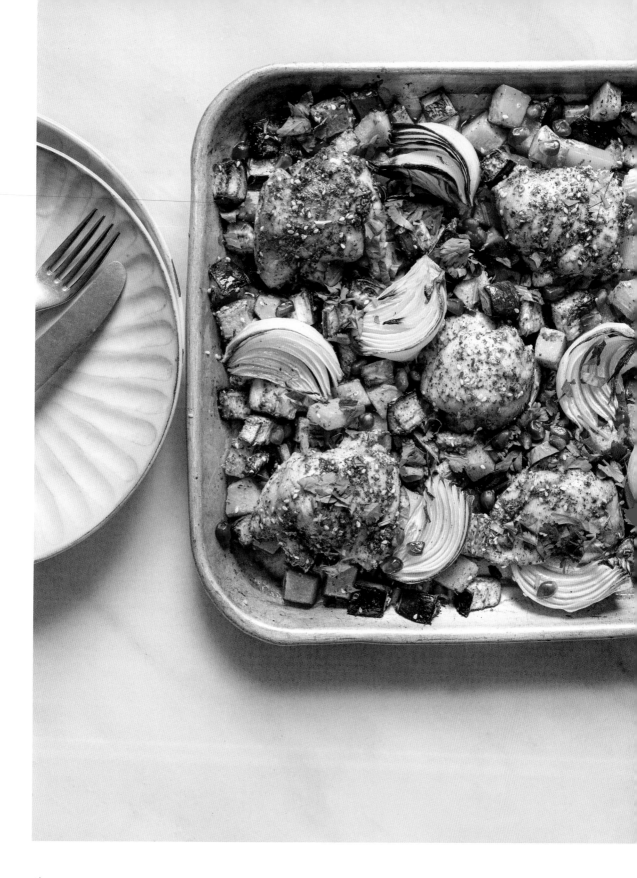

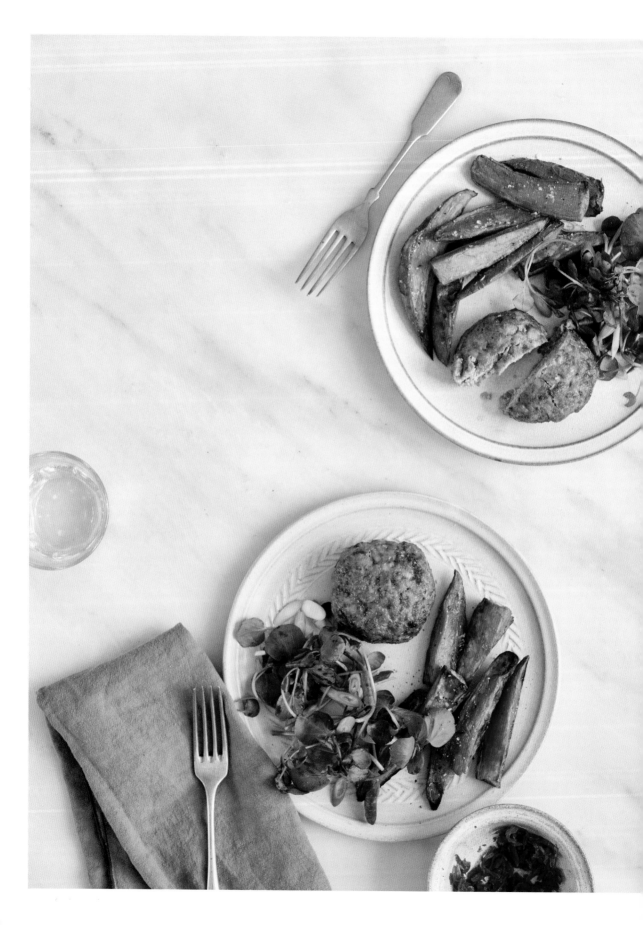

pea & chicken burgers

{Serves 4–6}
depending on their size

6 skinless, boneless
chicken thighs (500g)

150g frozen peas, thawed

2 spring onions,
roughly chopped

zest of ½ a lemon

2 tablespoons olive oil,
plus extra to drizzle

sea salt and freshly
ground black pepper

This is a real crowd-pleaser, and perfect if you are feeding the whole family, as kids seem to love these burgers. (Tried and approved by many in my house!) I make double the quantity and freeze half (once cooked) for a later date. I serve them with a side of simple steamed broccoli dressed with olive oil, and perhaps some quick potato wedges.

Preheat the oven to 240°C/220°C fan, and line a baking tray with baking parchment.

Put the chicken thighs, peas, spring onions, lemon zest and 2 tablespoons of olive oil into a food processor, add a sprinkle of salt and a decent grind of black pepper, and pulse until it looks well combined. Don't over-blend though, as you'll lose a bit of texture.

Using your hands, roughly shape the mixture into burgers. Place them on your lined baking tray, drizzle with a little olive oil and bake for approximately 25 to 30 minutes, or until well cooked through and lightly golden on top.

Serve hot.

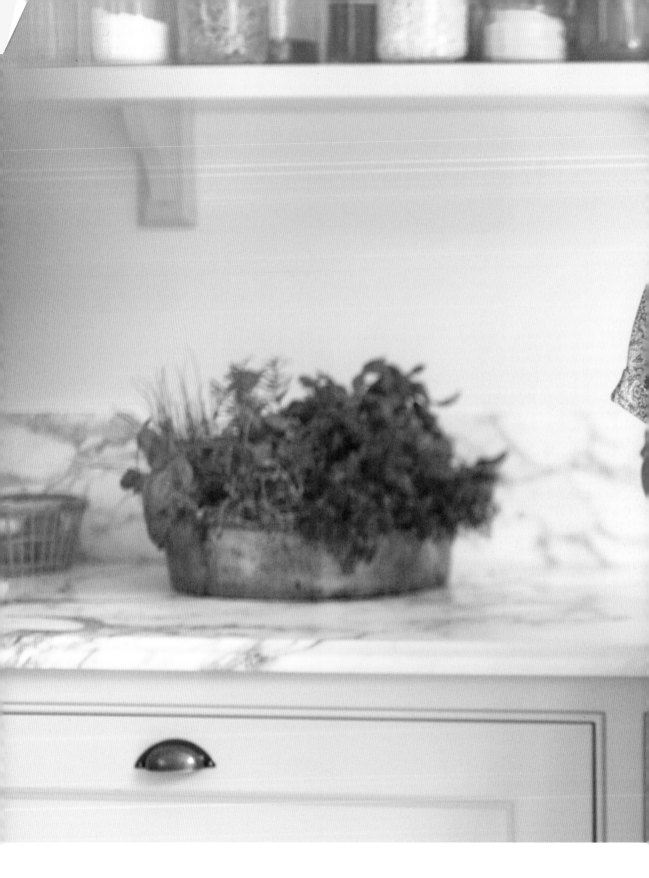

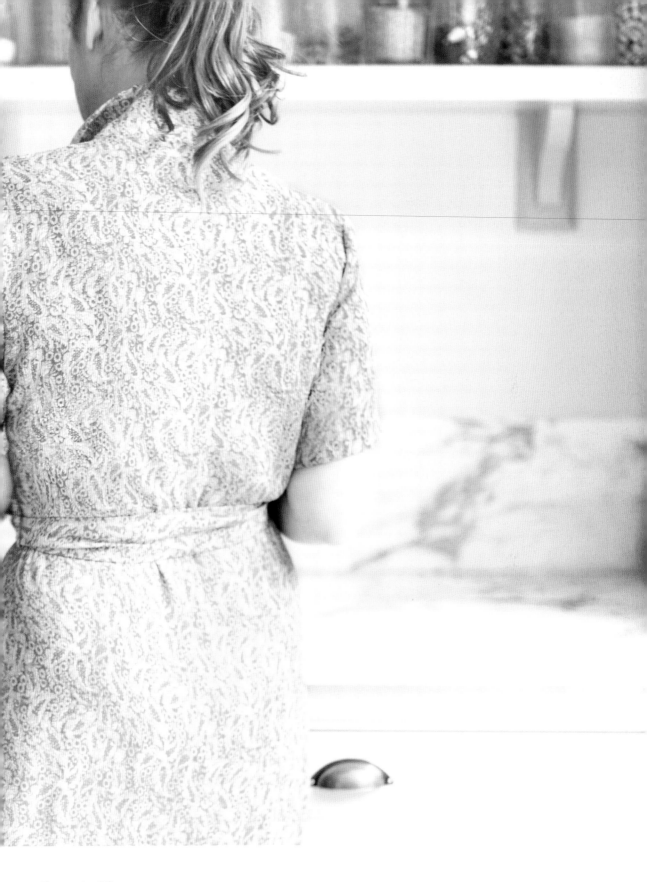

turkey & vegetable chilli

{Serves 8}

Chilli is such a useful recipe to have up your sleeve, and this version is packed full of vegetables and lean protein from the turkey mince, creating the basis of a very balanced meal. I serve it with some wilted greens, a little mashed avocado and chopped coriander, but if you're feeding hungry mouths, it works brilliantly spooned into jacket potatoes. It freezes well, which makes it a great recipe to batch cook, and children like it too if you omit the chilli. You can substitute beef mince or lentils for the turkey, change up the vegetables, and adjust the amount of chilli to your own taste preferences.

In a large wok, sauté the onions and garlic in a little olive oil for 10 to 15 minutes. Add the diced courgette, pepper and mushrooms, and cook for a few minutes, until softened. Then add the turkey mince, breaking it up with the back of a spoon. Sauté the whole lot together for 15 to 20 minutes, or until any water that is released from the meat and vegetables has evaporated.

Next, add the smoked paprika, cumin and chilli powder or fresh chillies, and stir well. Add the kidney beans, chopped tomatoes, water and tomato purée, along with a generous seasoning of salt and pepper. Stir, then simmer gently, uncovered, for 25 to 30 minutes or so, adding the spinach for the last 5 minutes (if using fresh spinach, just stir it through for 1 minute).

2 **onions**, peeled and diced

2 **large garlic cloves**, peeled and crushed (or 2 teaspoons garlic purée)

olive oil

2 **medium courgettes**, finely diced or grated

2 **red peppers**, deseeded and finely diced

200g **mushrooms**, finely diced

1kg **turkey mince** (I usually go for thigh meat)

2 teaspoons **smoked paprika**

2 teaspoons **ground cumin**

1 teaspoon **chilli powder**, or 1–2 **fresh chillies** (depending on how hot you like it!)

1 x 400g tin of **red kidney beans**, drained and rinsed

1 x 400g tin of **chopped tomatoes**

400ml **water**

4 tablespoons **tomato purée**

sea salt and freshly ground **black pepper**

3–4 blocks of **frozen spinach**, or 125g **baby leaf spinach**, roughly chopped

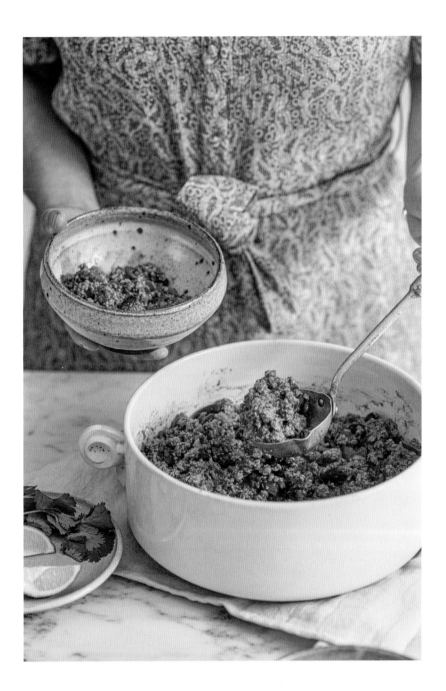

coconut lemon chicken

{Serves 6}

This has become my go-to summer entertaining dish. It tastes even better the next day so is ideal for preparing ahead. This can be made using chicken breasts, but I far prefer taking the time to roast a whole chicken – using a mixture of the white and dark meat is more economical, and creates a much more tender and juicy final dish. Plus you can use the leftover skin and bones to make a batch of chicken stock, which you can freeze or use for another recipe – freshly made stock will keep, covered, in the fridge for 3 days and in the freezer for 3 to 4 months.

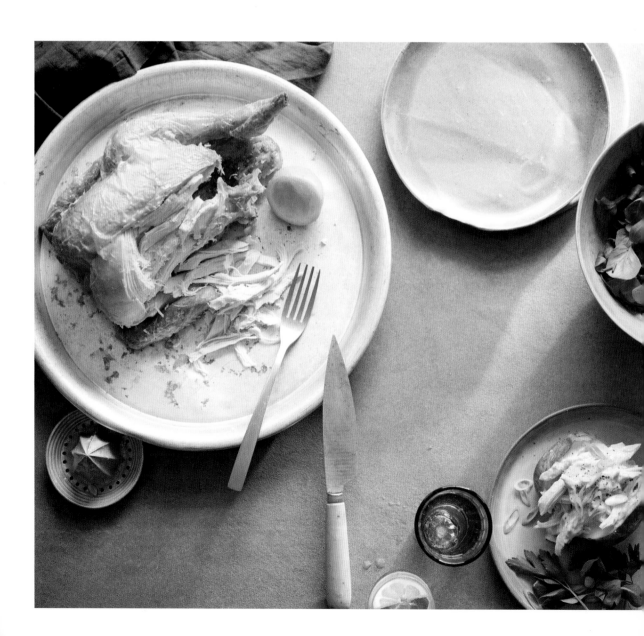

1 large chicken (approx. 1.8–2kg)

1 lemon, pricked all over with a knife

4 heaped tablespoons coconut yoghurt

100ml chicken stock (ideally the 'real deal', although at a push you could use a cube – just avoid adding much more salt)

2 spring onions, sliced

sea salt and freshly ground black pepper

To serve

1 bag of mixed salad leaves + fresh herbs of choice

6 jacket potatoes (optional)

Preheat the oven to 200°C/180°C fan.

Uncover and untruss the chicken (cut and remove any strings tying it up), and place it on a roasting tray. Place the pricked lemon inside the cavity and roast it whole for 1 to 1½ hours (or until cooked through and the juices run clear – use a meat thermometer if you are unsure, it should read 72°C in the thickest part of the chicken). If you are making jacket potatoes, pop them into the oven for the last 45 minutes.

Once cooked, remove the chicken from the oven and allow to cool thoroughly. When cool, remove all the meat from the bones, discarding the skin as you go. Whisk the coconut yoghurt, chicken stock and spring onions together. Taking the lemon from the centre of the chicken, cut it in half and squeeze out all the juice (straining it through a sieve helps avoid the pips going everywhere). Add the juice to the coconut yoghurt mixture.

Mix the chicken meat and the coconut sauce together in a bowl, add plenty of freshly ground black pepper and a little salt to taste, and leave to marinate for a few hours in the fridge until needed.

Serve with a herby green salad and baked jacket potatoes, if you like.

slow-cooked fennel, lemon, chicken & cannellini bean stew

{Serves 4–6}

Stews and casseroles are essential cooking if you need to keep things simple. I used to avoid them as I thought they were really hard and complicated. But once I got a slow cooker, this all changed and I now make them all year round. Fennel is up there with my top favourite vegetables and works very well in a stew. This is a summery, fragrant meal that is loved by everyone I serve it to, despite how effortless it is to make.

125ml chicken stock

125ml white wine

1 tablespoon Dijon mustard

1 teaspoon sea salt flakes, plus more for the chicken

1 lemon (peeler needed to remove some zest in strips)

1 onion, peeled and diced

6 large chicken thighs, skin removed

2 small fennel bulbs, stalks and fronds removed, bulbs cut lengthwise into thin wedges (approx. 600g)

2 sprigs of fresh thyme

200g tomatoes, roughly chopped (or tinned tomatoes, but fresh is better)

1 x 400g tin of cannellini beans, drained and rinsed

1 tablespoon extra virgin olive oil

10g fresh dill, chopped

In the crock of a slow cooker, blend together the chicken stock, white wine, mustard, salt, 3 strips of lemon zest and the juice of ½ the lemon, then add the onion.

Sprinkle the chicken all over with ½ teaspoon of sea salt and add it to the slow cooker along with the fennel, thyme and tomatoes. Cover and cook on the high heat setting for 4 hours.

Add the tinned cannellini beans, and cook on high for another 30 minutes.

Before serving, add the extra virgin olive oil and the juice of the remaining ½ lemon. Gently stir without breaking up the chicken pieces.

Serve sprinkled with chopped fresh dill.

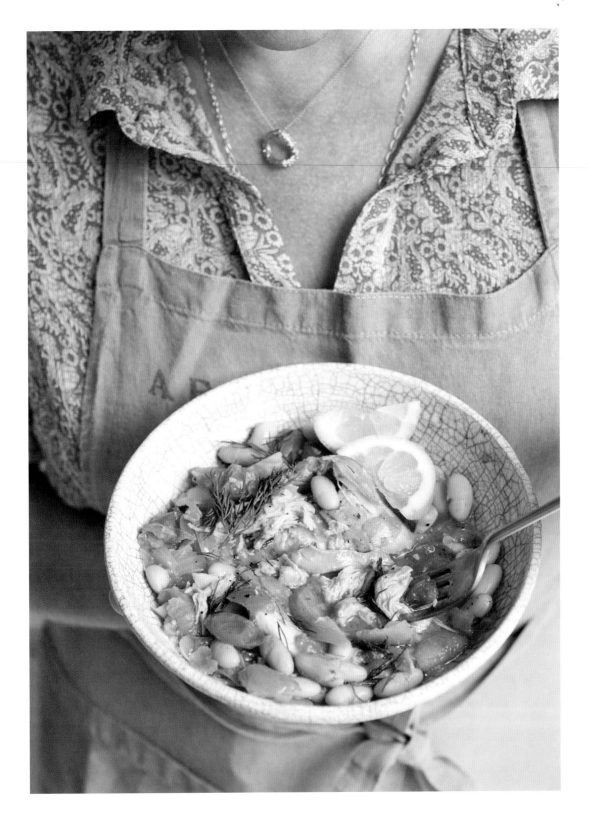

chicken pilaf

A one-pot recipe is always appealing to me and means more time doing the things I want to do, and less time washing up. I've fallen back in love with rice in the last couple of years and find this an intensely comforting dish. I'll often add mushrooms, courgettes or peppers to this while cooking to increase the vegetables, otherwise I serve it with a fresh and crisp green salad.

{Serves 4}

2 skinless, boneless chicken thighs (approx. 300g)

1 teaspoon sea salt

freshly ground black pepper

olive oil

1 onion, finely sliced

1 teaspoon ground cumin

200g brown rice (medium grain)

80g sultanas

2 teaspoons ground turmeric

1 unwaxed lemon

750ml chicken stock

40g pine nuts (or cashews)

25g fresh mint leaves, finely chopped

Season the chicken thighs with salt and pepper.

In a large heavy-based saucepan, heat 2 tablespoons of olive oil on a medium heat. Add the chicken and cook until brown. Remove from the pan and slice into thin strips, then set aside.

Add the onions and cumin to the same pan, and fry (stirring regularly) until the onions are lightly golden and tender.

Now add the rice, sultanas, turmeric, ½ teaspoon of ground black pepper and 3 strips of lemon zest (I just use a vegetable peeler to do this) and cook together for about a minute, until everything is slightly toasted and aromatic.

Next, carefully add the chicken stock, as it will splutter. Pop the chicken strips back into the pan and bring to a simmer. Cover with a tightly fitting lid wrapped in a tea towel, to prevent the steam from escaping. Reduce the heat to very low, and cook for 35 to 40 minutes, until all the liquid is absorbed and the rice is tender. Once cooked, set the pilaf aside, covered, for 10 minutes.

Toast the pine nuts or cashews in a dry pan, and keep shaking until they are lightly coloured. Don't take your eyes off them while doing this, as they tend to burn quickly! As soon as they are slightly golden, add a teaspoon of olive oil and a pinch of salt and mix well to coat.

Before serving, fluff the pilaf rice with a fork, then squeeze over the juice of ½ the lemon, and scatter over the chopped mint leaves and the pine or cashew nuts.

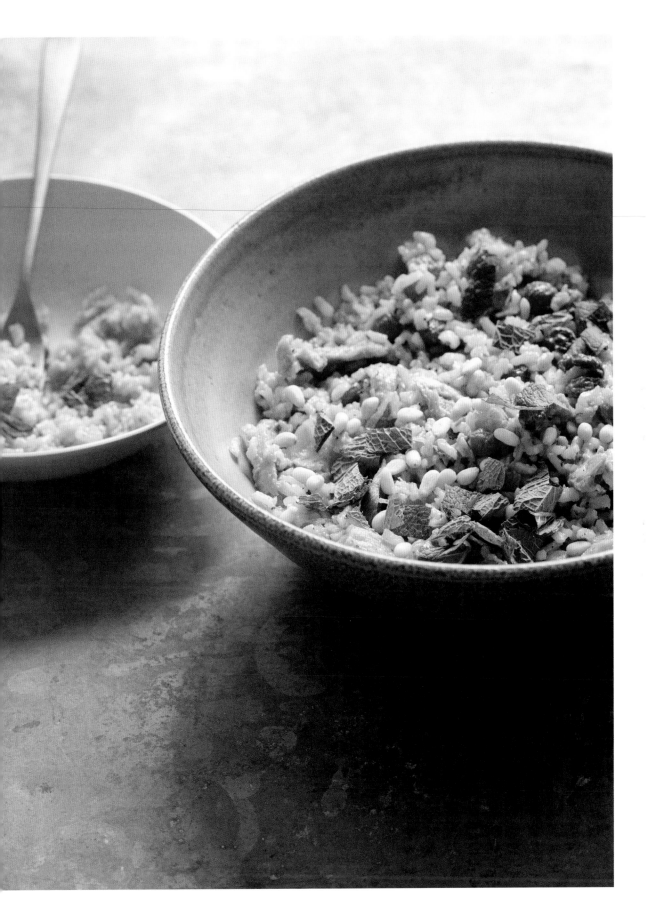

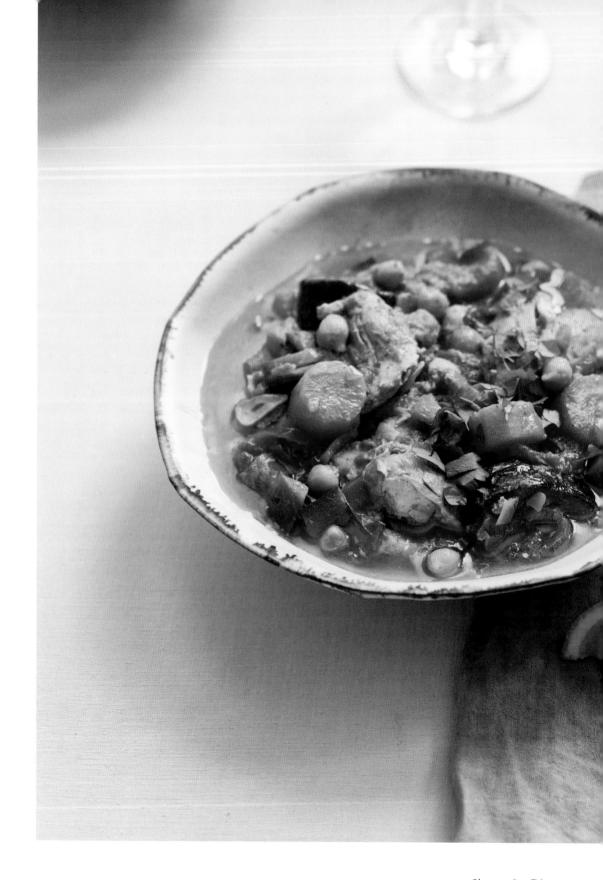

slow cooker summer chicken curry

{Serves 4}

A glut of summer vegetables on a chilly summer day became this glorious aromatic curry. I keep the spices mild if serving to children and add more later for grown-ups. This doesn't need rice or bread, just enjoy all of the vegetables. Leave out the chicken for a plant-based version and double the portion of chickpeas and add some toasted cashews or almonds to serve.

2 tablespoons coconut or olive oil

1 onion, peeled and finely diced

1 teaspoon salt, plus a little extra for the chicken

4 cloves of garlic, peeled and sliced

2 teaspoons minced fresh ginger

1 tablespoon ground coriander

1 teaspoon garam masala

1 teaspoon ground turmeric

4 chicken thighs on the bone, skin removed

1 bulb of fennel, finely sliced

1 aubergine, cubed

1 red pepper, deseeded and sliced

1 courgette, cut into thick slices

1 carrot, cut into thick slices

300g fresh tomatoes, diced

125ml chicken stock

1 x 400g tin of coconut milk

1 x 400g tin of chickpeas, drained and rinsed

juice of ½ a lemon

a small handful of fresh basil or coriander, chopped, to serve

Preheat your slow cooker to high. Heat the coconut or olive oil and add in the onions, salt, garlic, ginger, ground coriander, garam masala and turmeric and cook on maximum heat for 10 minutes with the lid on, until the onions have softened.

Sprinkle a pinch of salt over the chicken thighs and add to the pot with all the vegetables.

Pour the stock and coconut milk over the chicken and vegetables. Replace the lid.

Cook for 4 hours. Then add the chickpeas and cook for another 30 minutes without the lid.

Add the juice of ½ a lemon and some chopped fresh basil or coriander to serve.

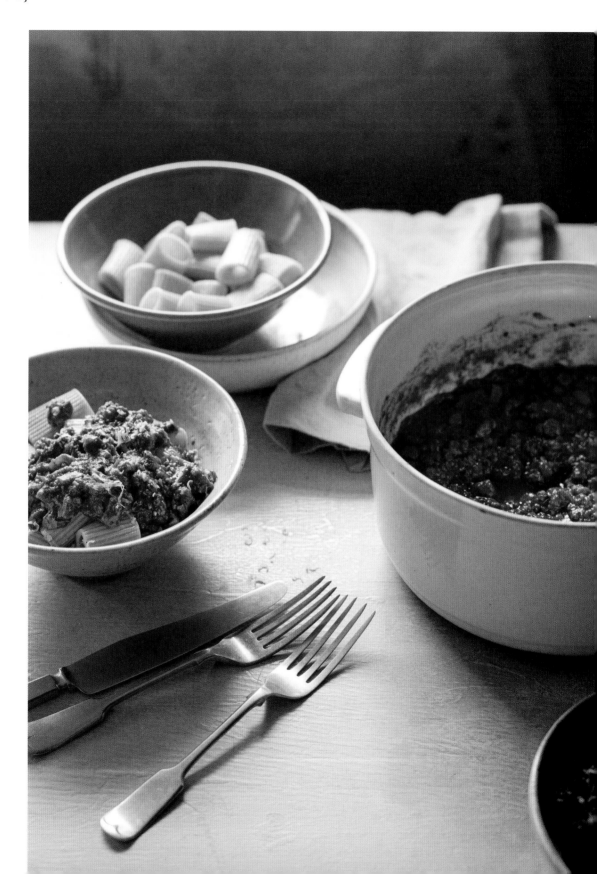

iron-rich ragù

I am not a huge fan of offal (and that is an understatement!). However, liver can be a fantastic source of dietary vitamins and minerals, especially iron. This ragù, which I made in batches and froze prior to the birth of my daughter, cleverly 'masks' the taste of the chicken livers, yet still delivers a nutritional punch. Perfect for restoring strength after an operation, illness or post-partum, or for anyone in need of a little extra iron. Note, I would not recommend this dish for pregnant women, as the vitamin A content in livers can be too high. This can be frozen in batches once cooked.

{Serves 8–10}

800g beef mince

1 courgette, diced

1 red pepper, deseeded and diced

a handful of mushrooms, diced

2 onions, peeled and diced

2 cloves of garlic, peeled and crushed

olive oil

300g organic chicken livers, finely chopped

1 glass of red wine

2 x 400g tins of chopped tomatoes

3–4 tablespoons tomato purée

1 teaspoon vegetable bouillon powder

sea salt and freshly ground black pepper

pasta of choice, to serve

Put the beef mince, courgettes, red peppers and mushrooms into a large slow cooker or casserole dish. Use the back of a wooden spoon to break up the mince a little.

Sauté the onions and garlic in a little olive oil until soft, then add the chopped livers and brown them well. Add this mixture to the casserole or slow cooker, along with the wine, tinned tomatoes, tomato purée and vegetable bouillon powder. Stir well.

In a slow cooker: cook on high (uncovered) for 4 to 6 hours, stirring occasionally.

In a casserole dish: cook at a very gentle simmer on the hob, covered, over a low heat for 2 to 3 hours, stirring occasionally (and adding a little extra water if it starts to look dry).

Season with salt and pepper before serving with your pasta of choice.

moussaka

{Serves 6 to 8}

Almost a complete all-in-one meal – I usually just add a pile of steamed greens or crispy salad. This recipe is perfect for cooking ahead, as it tastes even better the next day. It freezes well, making it a great one for batch cooking, and is popular with children too.

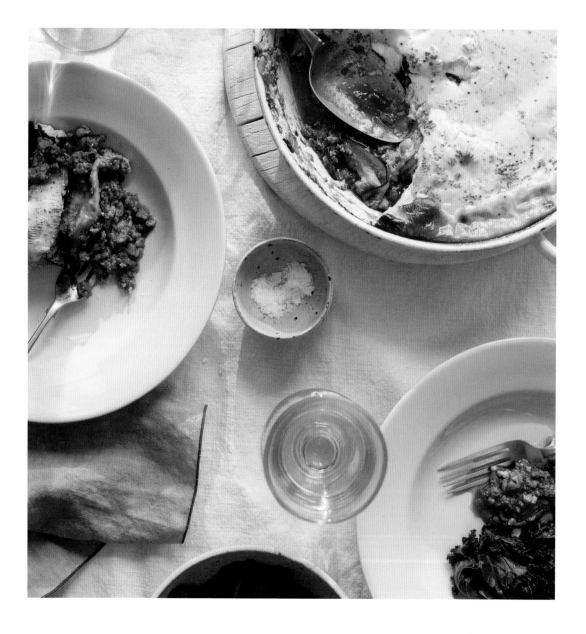

1 medium onion, peeled and diced (or 50g frozen onions)

2 large cloves of garlic, peeled and finely chopped (or 2 teaspoons garlic purée)

olive oil

1 large courgette, grated

800g lamb mince

2 teaspoons ground cumin

½ teaspoon ground cinnamon

1 x 400g tin of chopped tomatoes

1 medium bag of baby leaf spinach (approx. 125g)

sea salt and freshly ground black pepper

2 large aubergines, trimmed and sliced thinly lengthways

300g natural, unsweetened yoghurt (you can use cow's, sheep's or goat's milk yoghurt for this)

3 large eggs

50g feta

Sauté the onions and garlic in 1 tablespoon of olive oil in a large non-stick frying or sauté pan for 10 to 15 minutes, until softened. Add the grated courgette and the lamb mince and fry gently for 10 to 15 minutes or so, or until any water that has been released from the meat and vegetables has evaporated and the meat starts to stick a little to the pan.

Add the ground cumin and cinnamon and stir well. Then add the chopped tomatoes and half a tin of water (200ml). Stir in the baby spinach a handful at a time. Simmer for a further 10 minutes or so, then season to taste.

While the meat is cooking, preheat your grill to high.

Arrange the aubergine slices over a large baking sheet and drizzle with a little olive oil. You may need to do two batches (depending on the size of the slices and the size of your baking tray). Grill for 4 to 5 minutes each side, or until golden and soft. Once cooked, set to one side.

Whisk the yoghurt, eggs and feta together in a mixing bowl, and add a good grind of black pepper.

You are now ready to assemble! In a 20 x 25cm deep ovenproof baking dish, start with a meat layer, then cover with some aubergine slices, followed by more meat and more aubergines. Finally, top with the yoghurt mix, smoothing this over the top to cover the aubergines completely.

Bake at 200°C/180°C fan for 25 to 30 minutes, or until golden brown and bubbling. Leave to stand for 10 minutes before serving.

tip: I usually make 2 small trays, each serving roughly 3 to 4, and freeze the second for another day – I freeze when assembled, but not yet cooked.

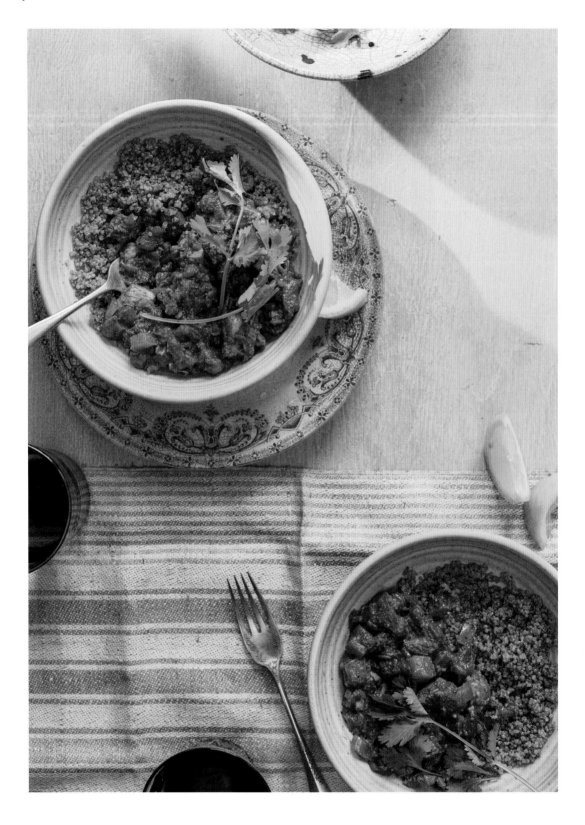

slow-cooked lamb & aubergine tagine

{Serves 8}

Quick to prepare, then slowly cooked, this tagine creates an unctuous, comforting, easily digestible bowl of goodness that can be cooked during the day, providing a perfect ready meal for when you get home. Serve with a pile of steamed greens drizzled with olive oil, and some quinoa.

900g diced lamb (large 3–4cm dice – ask for chopped leg or shoulder if you're buying from a butcher)

1 large aubergine, cut into 1cm cubes

1 red pepper, deseeded and diced

2 medium onions, peeled and diced

2 cloves of garlic, peeled and crushed

2 stalks of celery, diced

1 teaspoon ground coriander

2 teaspoons ground cumin

½ teaspoon ground cinnamon

1 level teaspoon sea salt

a good grind of black pepper

1 x 400g tin of chopped tomatoes, plus ½ tin (200ml) of water

1 tablespoon tomato purée

To serve

quinoa (optional)

Place all the ingredients in a slow cooker, and mix well together. Cook on medium for 6 hours (or for 7 to 8 hours on low).

To cook in the oven
Preheat your oven to 160°C/140°C fan.

Place all the ingredients in a heavy-bottomed casserole dish with a tight-fitting lid. Cook for 4 to 6 hours, until tender. Check every couple of hours to stop it cooking dry – if this happens, just add a little more water.

tip: I love the convenience of being able to put everything straight into the slow cooker, but if you have time, you can brown the lamb in a pan first for a better flavour.

slow cooker pulled pork with apple slaw

{Serves 6–8}

A winning dish for feeding a crowd. It does take a while to marinate and cook, but the preparation time is absolutely minimal and once it's done you can walk away. You will come back to perfectly cooked pork, just ready to be served. I love this in summer, served with a heap of apple coleslaw, a little grainy mustard and a salad. But is just as delicious in the autumn with roasted squash or pumpkin and a pile of steamed greens.

6 tablespoons olive oil

1 tablespoon smoked paprika

1 teaspoon grainy mustard

1 tablespoon Worcestershire sauce

3 cloves of garlic, peeled and crushed, or 2 teaspoons garlic purée

2kg shoulder of pork, skin and underlying fat removed

200ml stock (using a stock cube or bouillon powder is fine)

For the slaw

1 large eating apple, cored and grated

1 small or ½ a large green or red cabbage, stems removed and leaves finely sliced

4–5 medium carrots, peeled and grated

3–4 heaped tablespoons unsweetened natural yoghurt or coconut yoghurt

1 tablespoon apple cider vinegar

sea salt and freshly ground black pepper

Mix together the olive oil, smoked paprika, mustard, Worcestershire sauce and garlic, then rub this mixture all over the pork joint.

Ideally, allow it to marinate for a few hours (or overnight). However, if you don't have time for this, you can just put the pork straight into the slow cooker with the stock and start it cooking. Cook on the lowest setting for 8 hours.

Once cooked, remove the pork from the slow cooker, ditch any fatty bits, then, using two forks, pull the meat apart into shreds. Pile these on a serving dish and you're ready to go.

To cook in the oven
Preheat your oven to 160°C/140°C fan.

Place the marinated pork in a heavy-bottomed casserole dish, along with the stock. Cover with a tight-fitting lid. Cook for 4 to 6 hours, until falling apart when pushed with a fork. Check every couple of hours to stop it cooking dry – if this happens, just add a little more stock.

When cooked, finish preparing as above.

For the slaw
Mix all the ingredients together and season with salt and pepper to taste.

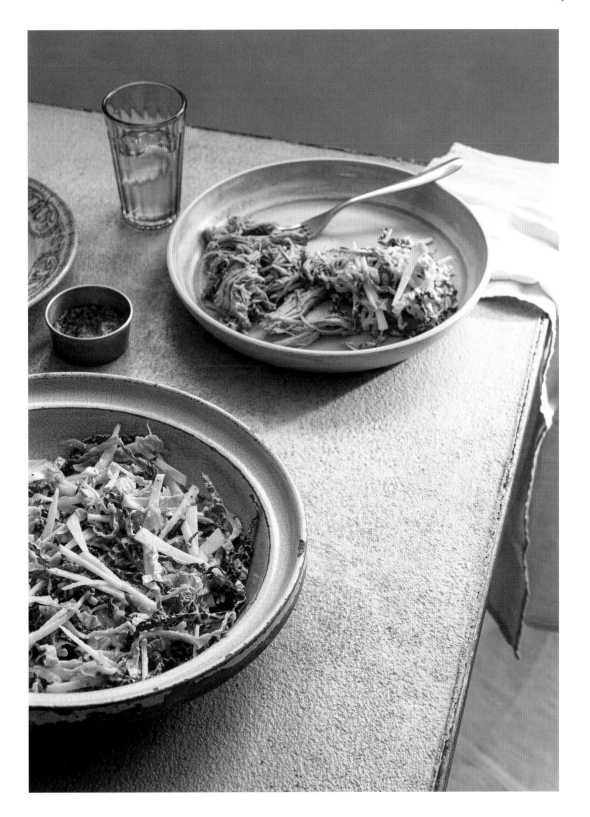

slow-cooked
beef brisket

{Serves 4}

*This is one of my go-to meals to serve
to friends and family on a wintery night
when I have very little time. It's wonderful
because it can all be made in advance and
the flavours get better. It also freezes well
so is handy for busy days.*

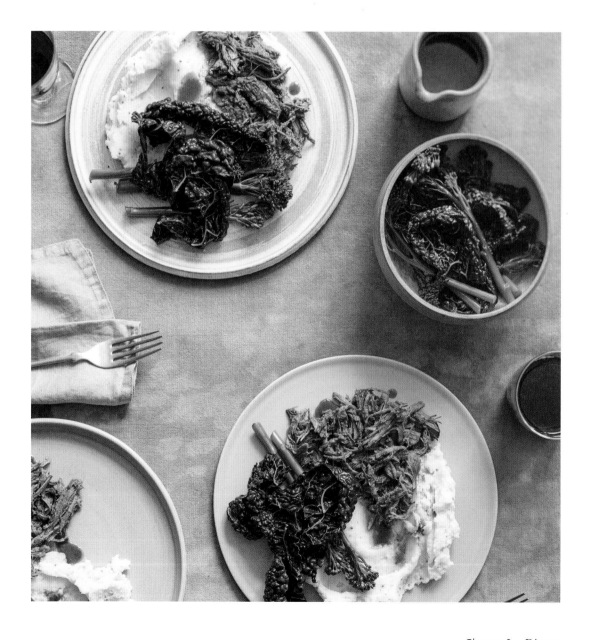

1.2kg beef brisket, rolled, boneless

1 whole head of garlic – cut in half, across the bulbous part (no need to peel)

2 red onions, peeled and halved

½ a bottle of red wine (375ml)

1 tablespoon stock powder, such as vegetable bouillon powder

3 tablespoons tomato purée

2–3 sprigs of woody herbs, such as thyme, rosemary or bay

freshly ground black pepper

To serve

1.5kg potatoes, peeled and cut into chunks

3 tablespoons olive oil

150–200ml milk of your choice

wholegrain mustard or grated nutmeg

sea salt

400g tenderstem broccoli, cavolo nero, or other greens you like

Place the beef brisket in a slow cooker, and add the garlic and onions around the sides. Add the red wine, stock powder, tomato purée, herbs and a generous grind of black pepper.

Top up with enough boiling water (it helps bring the temperature up quicker) to come two-thirds of the way up the beef brisket. Put the lid on and cook on low for 6 to 10 hours. When cooked, the meat should be completely falling apart and incredibly tender.

When the beef is nearly ready, cook the potatoes for 15 to 20 minutes in boiling water until tender. Drain, then mash with the olive oil, milk, a little mustard or nutmeg, and a pinch of salt and pepper, until smooth. Set aside and keep warm.

Remove the beef from the slow cooker and place on a serving dish. Strain the cooking liquid through a sieve into a pan and simmer for a few minutes to reduce, then drizzle a few spoonfuls over the top of the meat.

While the sauce is reducing, steam the greens for 3 to 4 minutes. Serve the beef with the mash and the steamed broccoli.

To cook in the oven

Put the ingredients into a heavy casserole with a tight-fitting lid and top up with enough boiling water to come two-thirds of the way up the beef brisket. Cover everything with a couple of layers of baking parchment, then put the lid on top. Cook at 140°C/120°C fan for 6 hours, or until the meat is falling apart. Check halfway through to ensure that there is still enough liquid, adding a little extra water if necessary, as you don't want it to cook dry.

If you have leftover beef, turn to page 103 for the beef and rocket salad.

lamb chops with spinach & white bean purée & greens

{Serves 2}

There is nothing wrong with eating mashed potato but I try, where I can, to diversify my food selections. White beans make a wonderful, creamy purée that contains a different range of nutrients than potatoes. It is therefore not better, just different, which is a good thing. Wherever you can, try to increase the variety of foods instead of sticking to the same few. This is traditional comfort food to fill and nourish you and can be on the table in under 15 minutes.

4 lamb chops

1 tablespoon olive oil

1 teaspoon ground cumin

sea salt and freshly ground black pepper

For the bean purée

100ml water

½ an onion, sliced

1 x 400g tin of butter beans, drained and rinsed

2 handfuls of baby leaf spinach

2 handfuls of watercress

juice of ½ a lemon

Put the lamb chops into a bowl with the olive oil and cumin, and season with salt and pepper. Allow to marinate for at least 5 minutes, the longer the better (if marinating for longer than 5 minutes, leave it in the fridge).

When ready to cook, heat a non-stick frying pan and, once hot, put in the lamb chops. Cook on a medium-high heat for 4 minutes, then turn them over and cook for a further 2 minutes. If you prefer them more well done, simply cook them for longer. Leave to rest in a bowl for a few minutes before serving.

To make the purée, put the water and sliced onion into a saucepan. Bring to a simmer and cook for 5 minutes, until the onion is soft. Add the beans and cook for another 2 minutes, until the beans have softened. Top up with water if it looks dry. Transfer to a blender and blend until creamy, adding a splash of cold water if needed.

Return the purée to the pan and season with salt and pepper. Add the spinach and stir until it wilts.

Serve the lamb chops with the bean and spinach purée and a handful of watercress, dressed with lemon juice.

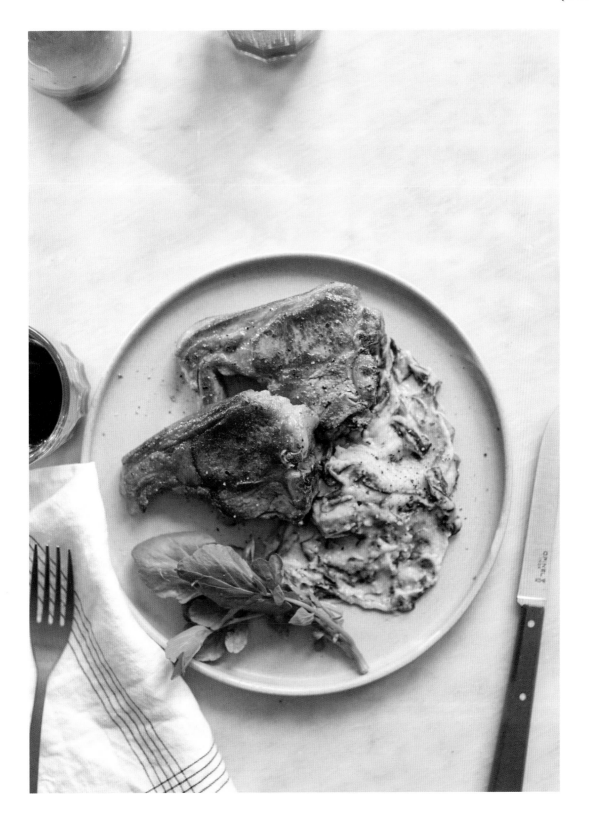

steak, crispy new potatoes, roasted tomatoes & sugar snap peas

{Serves 2}

Every once in a while I really enjoy a good steak. I am increasingly conscious of where I buy meat from due to ethical and environmental concerns, so when I do indulge, I go all-in and thoroughly enjoy.

250g cherry tomatoes, halved

2 tablespoons olive oil

1 tablespoon balsamic vinegar

sea salt and freshly ground black pepper

5 basil leaves, torn

200g baby new potatoes, washed and halved (but no need to peel)

2 thin-cut beef steaks (or minute steaks)

150g sugar snap peas

Preheat the oven to 220°C/200°C fan.

Line a baking tray with baking parchment. Arrange the halved tomatoes on a baking tray, then drizzle with 1 tablespoon of olive oil and the balsamic vinegar, then season with salt and pepper. Roast in the oven for 20 minutes. When done, remove from the oven and stir in the basil.

While the tomatoes are cooking, steam the halved new potatoes for about 15 minutes.

Rub the steaks with 1 tablespoon of olive oil, salt and pepper and fry in a hot pan for just a minute each side. Leave to rest in a bowl. Wipe out the pan and return it to the heat.

Tip the steamed potatoes into the frying pan and sprinkle with salt. Fry for 5 minutes on a medium-high heat, until golden.

Put the sugar snap peas into a bowl and cover with boiling water. Leave them for a minute until tender, then drain.

Divide the steaks, potatoes, tomatoes and peas between two plates, and serve.

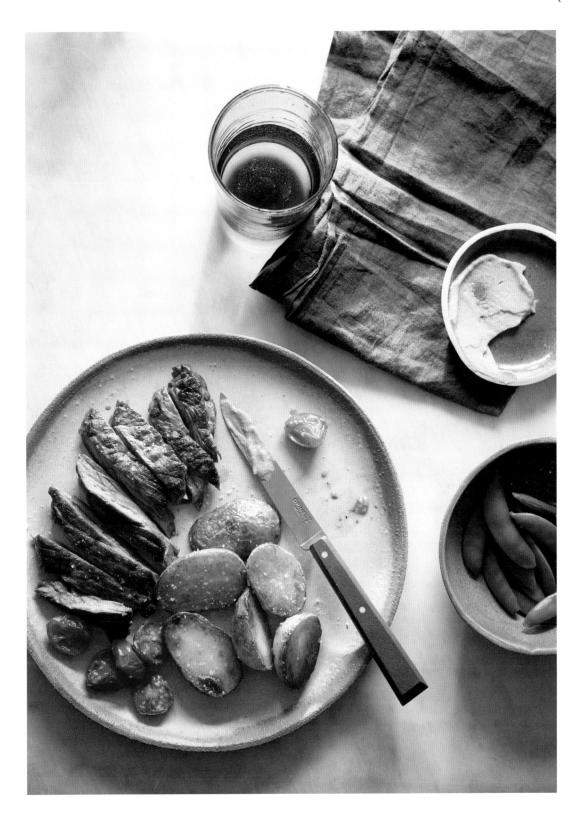

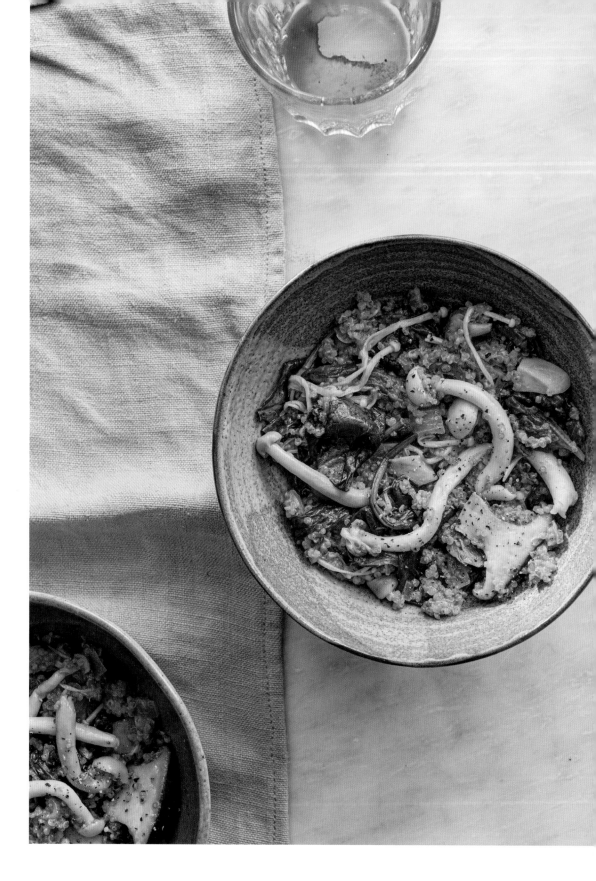

garlic mushroom quinoa risotto

Midwinter comfort food and much faster to cook than rice-based risotto. If you are strapped for time, use pre-cooked quinoa from a packet, but reduce the amount of stock you use – just a splash is all you'll need to prevent the mixture from tasting dry.

{Serves 2}

25g dried porcini mushrooms

1 onion, peeled and diced

olive oil

3 cloves of garlic, peeled and crushed

½ a punnet (approx. 175g) of chestnut mushrooms, diced (or wild mushrooms if you can get them)

150g quinoa, dried (or a 250g pouch of pre-cooked quinoa)

2 handfuls of baby leaf spinach

2 tablespoons coconut yoghurt/natural yoghurt

sea salt and freshly ground black pepper

Soak the porcini mushrooms in 700ml of boiling water.

In a large saucepan, sauté the onions in 2 tablespoons of olive oil until soft. Drain the porcini mushrooms, retaining the soaking liquid, and add the rehydrated mushrooms to the pan together with the garlic and the fresh mushrooms. Cook for a further 5 minutes.

Add the quinoa, and stir well. Pour over enough of the mushroom soaking liquid to just cover the quinoa. Bring to a gentle simmer. (If using pre-cooked quinoa, add 250ml of the mushroom soaking liquid, bring to a simmer, add the spinach and wilt for a minute, then remove from the heat and stir in the yoghurt.)

Cook for 20 to 30 minutes, or until the quinoa is cooked through, but still has some bite. You might need to add some more of the mushroom 'stock' if it is starting to look dry.

Right at the end of cooking, stir in the spinach and finally the yoghurt. Adjust the seasoning to taste before serving.

my weekly 'bottom of the fridge' vegetable stew

{Serves 4}

Every week I make a simple stew to use up the vegetables that are left over in my fridge. I then split this stew into several portions and serve some with butter beans or chickpeas, some with pasta, some with quinoa, and blend some to freeze for soups or sauces another time. You really can adapt this basic recipe to use up what vegetables you have. It can either be made in a slow cooker or a heavy-based, lidded casserole pan.

2 tablespoons olive oil

½ an onion, peeled and sliced

1 teaspoon sea salt

2 cloves of garlic, peeled and thinly sliced

3 celery stalks, cut into small slices

3 sprigs of fresh thyme

1 bay leaf

125ml white wine

1 aubergine, diced

200g mushrooms, sliced

1 fennel bulb, thinly sliced

250ml chicken or vegetable stock

250ml passata

6 cherry tomatoes, halved

1 teaspoon red wine vinegar

2 tablespoons extra virgin olive oil

freshly ground black pepper

fresh marjoram (optional)

Heat the olive oil in a large, non-stick frying pan over a medium heat. Add the onion slices and the salt and fry for 5 minutes, stirring regularly. Then add the garlic and keep frying until soft. Add the celery, thyme and bay leaf and fry for another minute. Then add the white wine and cook until it has all evaporated.

Transfer to a slow cooker, and add the diced aubergine, sliced mushrooms and fennel. Pour over the stock and passata, then cover and cook on high for 3 hours.

Alternatively, cook in a heavy-bottomed pan on the stove top, covered, for 50 minutes on a slow simmer. Stir occasionally to help stop the bottom catching.

Before serving, add the halved cherry tomatoes, a teaspoon of red wine vinegar, 2 tablespoons of extra virgin olive oil, some freshly ground black pepper and a sprinkling of fresh marjoram (if using). This really freshens the flavour.

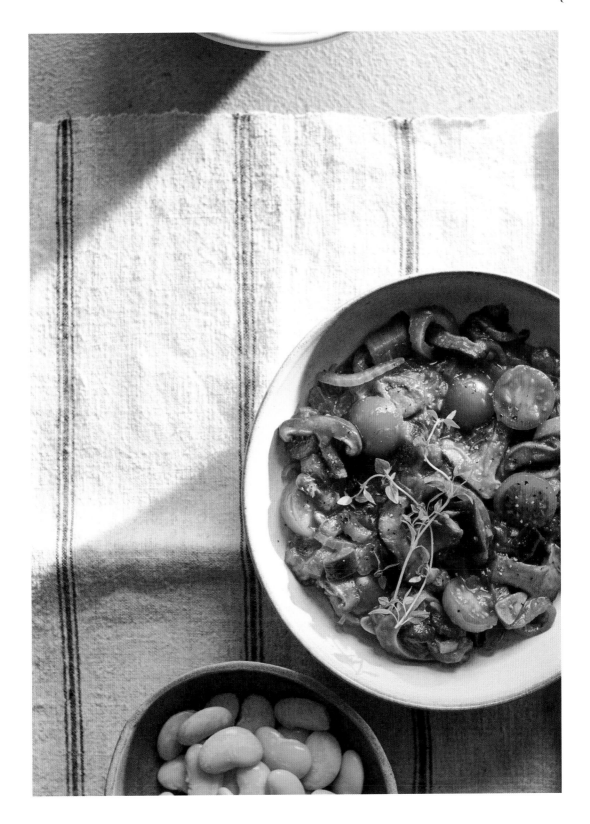

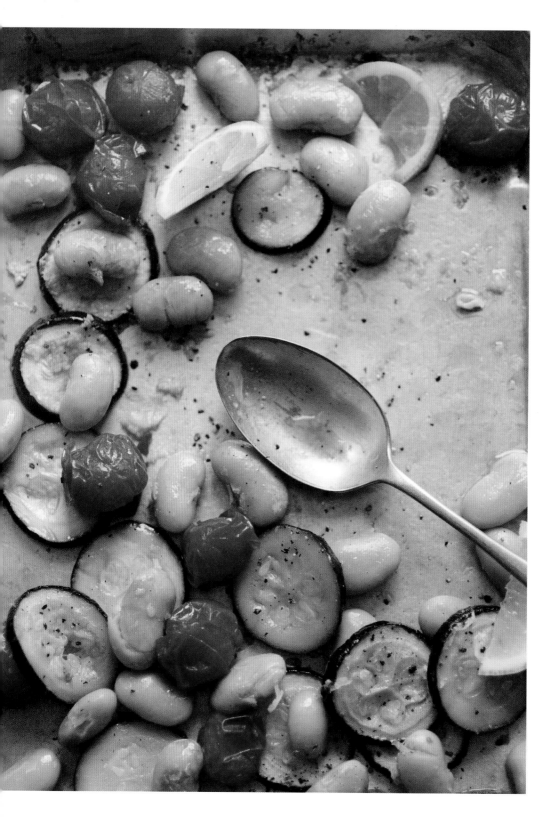

pan-fried garlic & lemon butter beans
(vegan)

{Serves 2}

Fresh, nutritious, filling and quick. You can easily double the quantities given if you are cooking for friends or would like to have some leftovers – which are great for lunch the next day with some salad and crumbled feta.

2 cloves of garlic, peeled and crushed

2 tablespoons olive oil

1 courgette, sliced into ½cm rounds

300g cherry tomatoes

1 x 400g tin of butter beans, drained and rinsed

½ an unwaxed lemon

a pinch of sea salt flakes

5 fresh basil leaves, torn

freshly ground black pepper

Sauté the garlic in a tablespoon of olive oil in a shallow pan or casserole dish. Add the courgettes and tomatoes and stir until they start to soften.

Add the butter beans and stir to gently warm them through.

Add the grated zest of ¼ of the lemon, a tablespoon or so of lemon juice, a pinch of sea salt flakes, the remaining tablespoon of olive oil and some fresh basil leaves. Top with a good grind of black pepper.

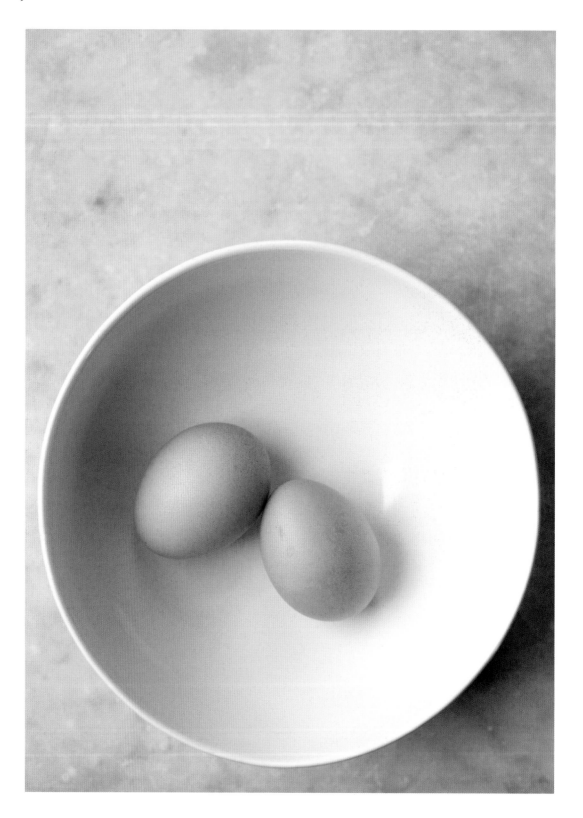

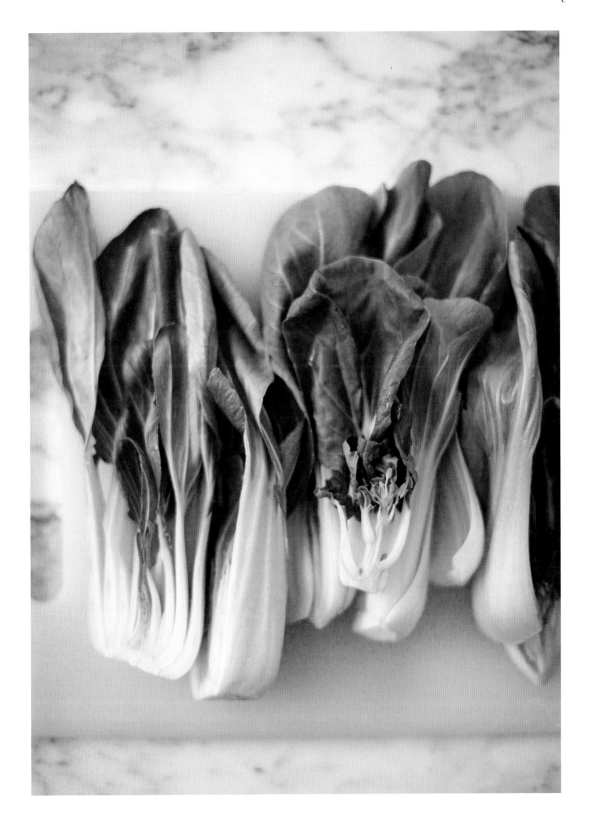

ginger greens & fried egg

{Serves 2}

A fried egg is such a simple staple but is often dismissed as unhealthy. However, add some greens to it and a little ginger and spice and we have a fine meal. For a plant-based version I'd add cooked quinoa, brown rice or lentils with toasted cashew nuts. Every time I see this recipe, I want to make and eat it instantly.

60g pak choi, leaves kept whole (just pull or chop them off the stem)

60g spinach

60g broccoli

½ teaspoon cumin seeds

2 teaspoons olive oil

5g fresh ginger, peeled and finely diced

1 or 2 anchovies, finely chopped

1 teaspoon coconut oil or olive oil

2 eggs

sea salt flakes

a sprinkling of chilli flakes

Wash the greens and cut the broccoli into small florets.

Heat a large, lidded non-stick frying pan on a medium heat. Once warm, put in the cumin seeds and toast them, regularly shaking the pan, for 2 minutes. Add the olive oil and the diced ginger, fry for a minute, then add the anchovies.

Add the greens (they should still be a little wet from being washed), give a little stir to coat them with the ginger and anchovies, and cover the pan. Cook until wilted (2 to 4 minutes, depending on taste). Remove the vegetables from the pan with a slotted spoon or tongs, and place on a clean plate.

Wipe out the pan and put in the coconut oil. Wait until it is very hot before cracking in the eggs. Add a sprinkling of salt and cook to your liking.

Place the eggs on top of the greens and add a sprinkling of chilli flakes.

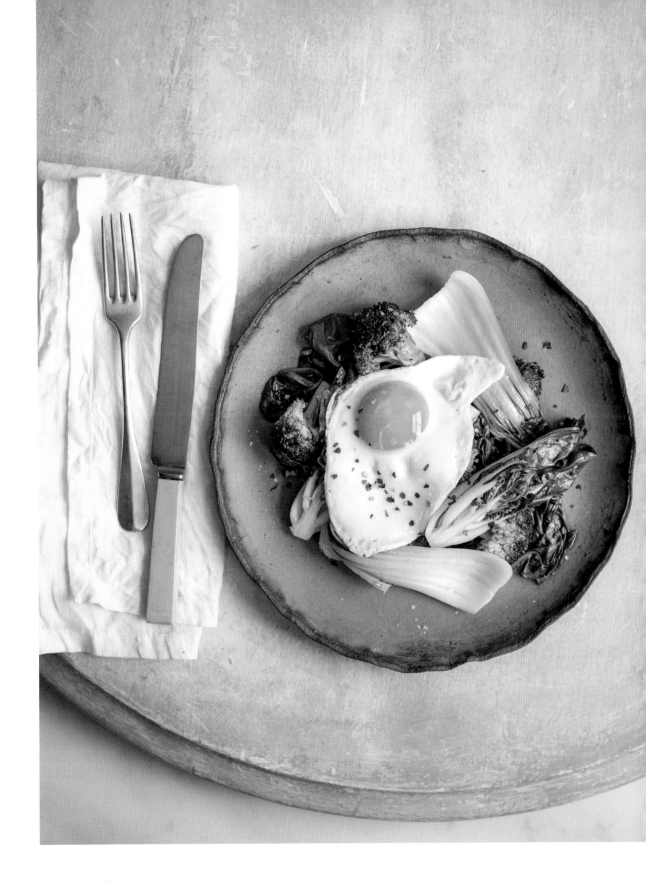

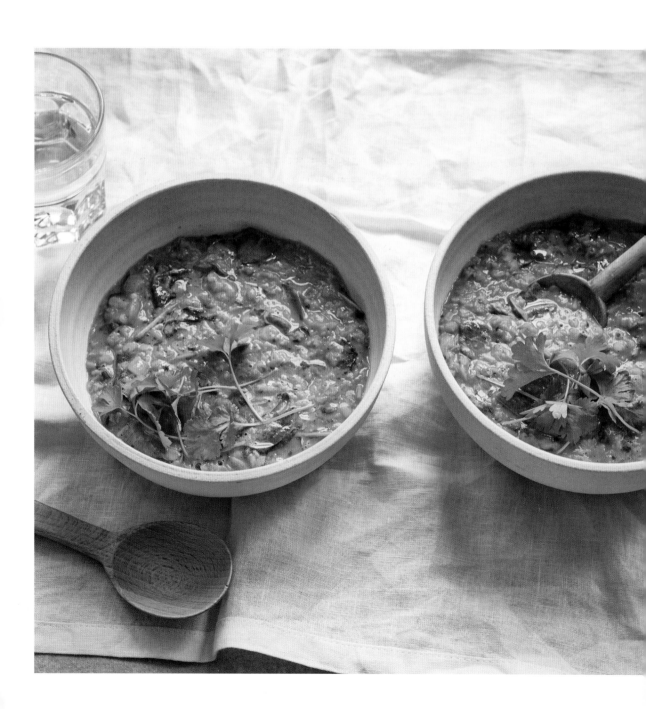

lazy dahl
(vegan)

{Serves 2}

I call it 'lazy' because I'll sometimes use frozen chopped onions, garlic, ginger and chilli, and skip the toasting of the spices (just substituting an equivalent amount of ground spices). It does save time and reduce all of the chopping. However, using fresh ingredients and taking that little bit of extra time really does produce better flavour, so I'll leave it with you to decide. It freezes well.

½ teaspoon cumin seeds

½ teaspoon coriander seeds

½ teaspoon mustard seeds

2 teaspoons coconut oil

1 onion, peeled and diced

3 cloves of garlic, peeled and finely chopped

1 tablespoon grated fresh ginger

1 red chilli, deseeded and finely chopped

2 teaspoons ground turmeric

1 teaspoon garam masala

200g dried red lentils, rinsed until the water runs clear, and drained

1 x 400g tin of coconut milk

500ml vegetable stock

sea salt and freshly ground black pepper

2 handfuls of washed fresh spinach or 2 blocks of frozen

juice of ½ a lemon

a handful of fresh coriander leaves

Heat a large pan over a medium heat and gently toast the cumin, coriander and mustard seeds for 2 to 3 minutes, until the mustard seeds start to pop. Tip them out of the pan, and then lightly grind in a pestle and mortar or spice grinder.

Put the coconut oil into the hot pan, then add the onion with a pinch of salt and cook gently for 5 minutes over a low heat. Add the garlic, ginger and chilli and cook for a further few minutes. Add the freshly ground spices, along with the turmeric and garam masala, and cook for 1 minute.

Finally, add the lentils, coconut milk and vegetable stock, and stir to combine. Bring to the boil, then reduce to a simmer. Cook on a low heat for 10 minutes with the lid on, then 10 minutes with the cover off to allow it to thicken. Taste and season with salt and pepper.

Just before serving, add the spinach and stir until it wilts, then squeeze in the lemon juice and top with fresh coriander leaves.

stir-fried veggies & tofu
(vegan)

{Serves 1}

Stir-fries are a go-to quick and easy meal. This vegan version is a colourful feast, with added protein from the tofu and peanuts. Use whichever vegetables you have available. Just multiply the ingredients list by the number of people you are serving.

1 tablespoon tamari or soy sauce

1 teaspoon rice vinegar

1 teaspoon maple syrup or honey

1 teaspoon toasted sesame oil

60g uncooked rice noodles

150g tofu, cubed into bite-size pieces

¼ teaspoon sea salt

¼ teaspoon smoked paprika or chipotle chilli powder

2 tablespoons olive oil

1 red chilli, deseeded and finely sliced

1 clove of garlic, peeled and finely sliced

1 red or yellow pepper, deseeded and sliced

125g tenderstem broccoli

a small handful of fresh chives, finely chopped

20g roasted and salted peanuts, roughly chopped

Mix together the tamari, vinegar, maple syrup and sesame oil in a serving bowl.

Cook the noodles in boiling water according to the packet instructions, then drain and rinse well. Add to the serving bowl and mix with the dressing.

Make sure the cubes of tofu are dry (I use kitchen paper for this). Mix them with the salt and smoked paprika.

Heat a non-stick frying pan over a medium heat. Once warm, add 1 tablespoon of olive oil. Add the cubes of tofu and fry for a couple of minutes on each side, until crisp. Resist the urge to stir too much or they may break apart! Once browned and crispy, put aside on a plate.

Add the remaining oil to the pan, followed by the chilli and garlic. Fry for a short minute, then add the pepper strips and broccoli and cook until softened, about 5 minutes.

Tip the veg and tofu into the noodles, and mix together. Sprinkle with the chives and peanuts to serve.

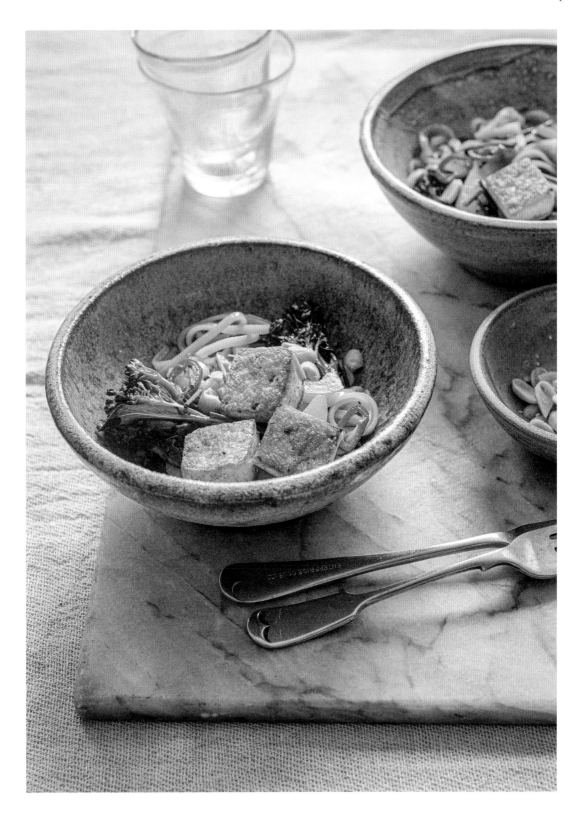

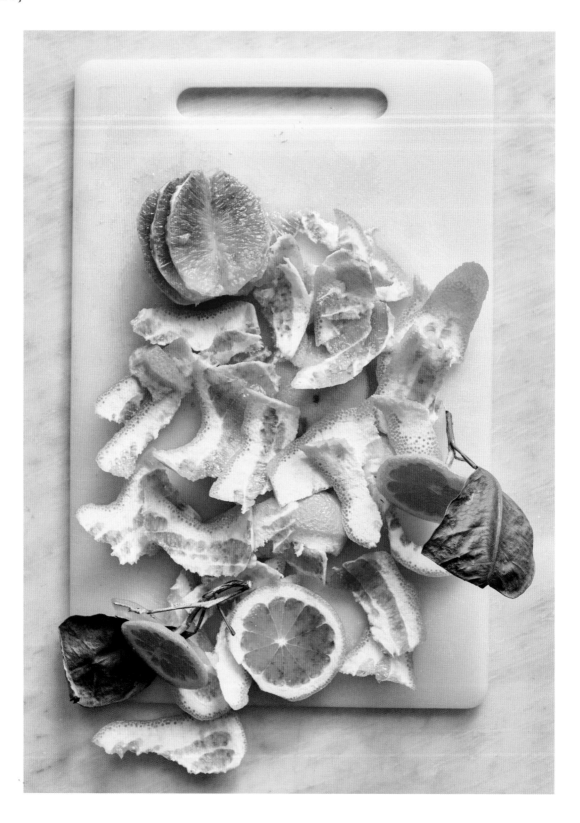

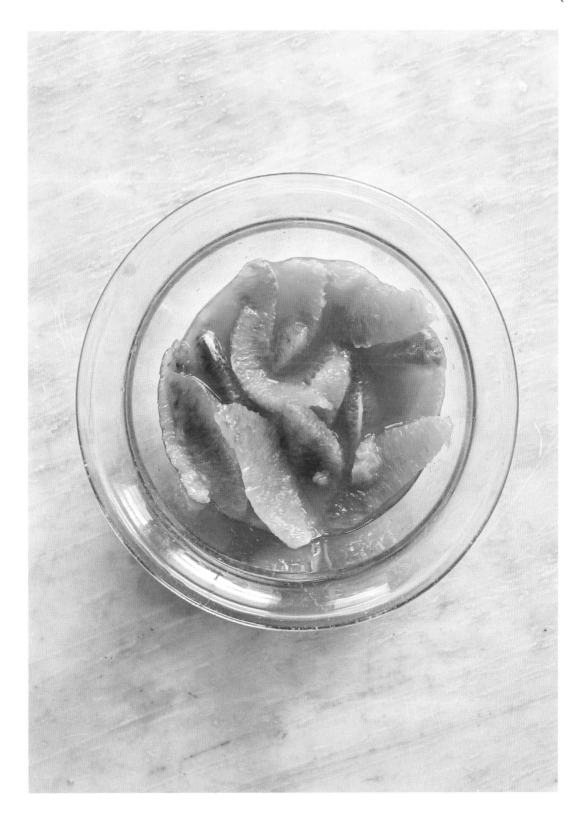

one-tray roasted winter salad

(vegan)

{Serves 2}

Roasted salads are a total game-changer for me. However sceptical you may be – just give it a go. The textures soften and the flavours enhance. It's really no more complicated than making a 'standard' salad. It also is delicious cold the next day.

1 small butternut squash,* peeled, deseeded and cut into chunks

2 small red onions, peeled and cut into quarters

1 x 400g tin of chickpeas, drained and rinsed

2 handfuls of kale, tough stalks removed first, sliced into ribbons

a small handful of hazelnuts (approx. 30g)

1 orange, peeled and torn or sliced into segments

sea salt and freshly ground black pepper

For the dressing

2 tablespoons olive oil

2 tablespoons balsamic vinegar

1 teaspoon Dijon mustard

a pinch of sea salt

Preheat the oven to 200°C/180°C fan.

Whisk together all the dressing ingredients until emulsified and smooth.

Tumble the butternut squash chunks, red onions and chickpeas on to a roasting tray, and pour over half the dressing, turning it all over a few times to make sure everything is well coated. Roast for 30 to 35 minutes, or until the squash is tender and cooked through.

Add the sliced kale to the roasting tray, along with the rest of the dressing, and mix well. Sprinkle with the hazelnuts. Roast for a further 5 to 7 minutes, until the kale is a little wilted. Take care it doesn't burn.

Divide between two bowls, allow to cool slightly, then top with the orange segments and season with salt and pepper to taste.

*

tip: Sweet potato would also work well.

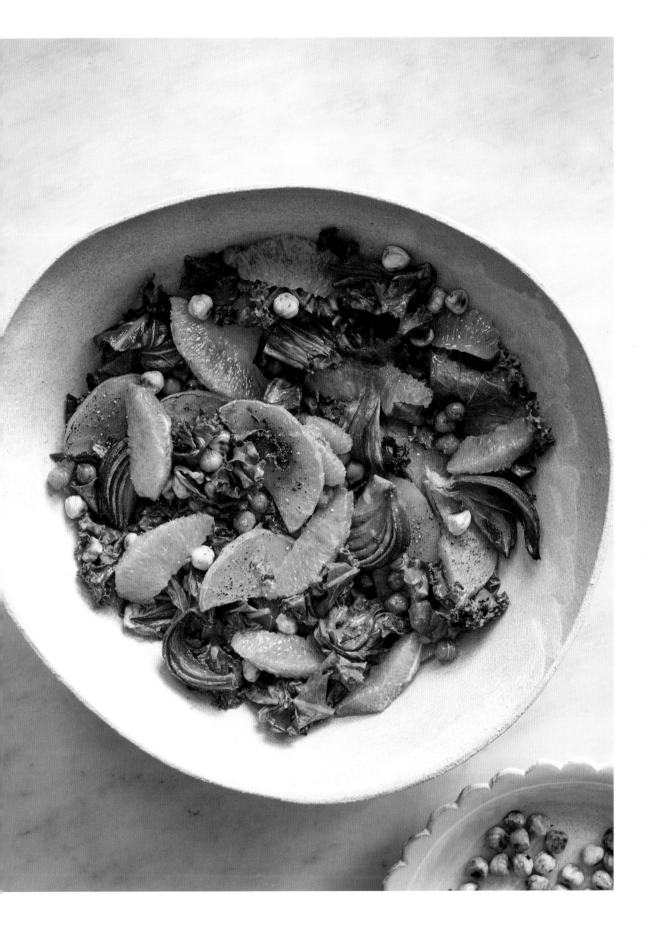

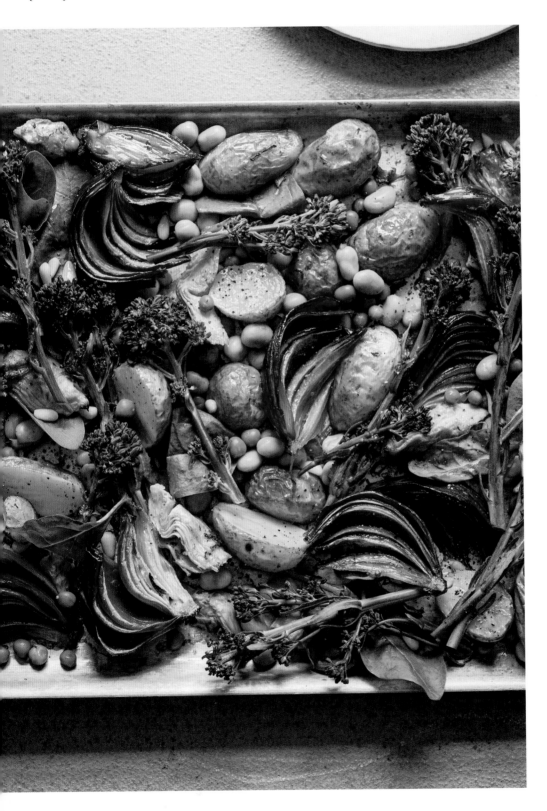

one-tray roasted summer salad

(vegan)

{Serves 2}

Roasting a salad? Yes, I thought it was nuts too. But then I tried it and fell in love! Pile various salad ingredients on to a baking tray, cover them in the dressing and roast them until cooked and a little crispy. One tray to wash up and a warm, colourful, elaborate meal that is just that little bit more exciting than a regular salad of lettuce, cucumber and tomato. It is also just as good eaten cold the next day (so I'd recommend you make enough for lunch too).

a generous handful (200g) of new potatoes, halved

2 red onions or shallots, peeled, cut into quarters

1 jar of artichoke hearts, drained (optional)

1 small head of broccoli, cut into small florets (or use sprouting broccoli)

a small handful of pine nuts (approx. 30g)

2 big handfuls of frozen broad beans or peas (approx. 150g)

1 big handful of baby leaf spinach

sea salt and freshly ground black pepper

For the dressing

2 tablespoons olive oil

zest of ½ a lemon

2 tablespoons lemon juice

1 teaspoon Dijon mustard

a pinch of sea salt

Preheat the oven to 200°C/180°C fan.

Whisk together all the dressing ingredients until emulsified and smooth.

Tumble the new potatoes, onions and artichokes (if using) on to a roasting tray. Mix through half the dressing. Roast for 35 to 40 minutes, until the potatoes are browned and cooked all the way through (the cooking time will vary depending on the size of the potatoes).

Add the broccoli, pine nuts, broad beans/peas and the rest of the dressing to the tray. Roast for a further 5 to 7 minutes, until the broccoli has just softened.

Remove the tray from the oven and stir through the spinach. It will wilt in the latent heat of the tray.

Divide between two bowls, and season with salt and pepper. You might want to add another squeeze of lemon.

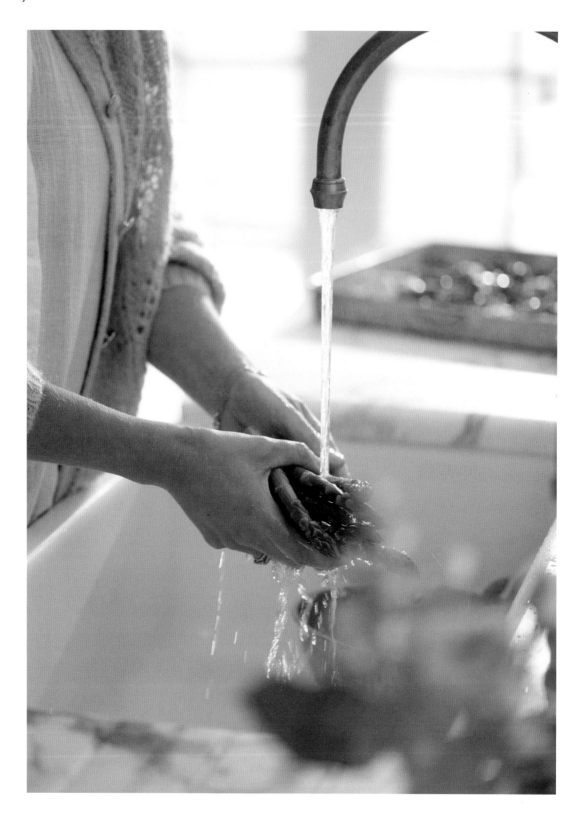

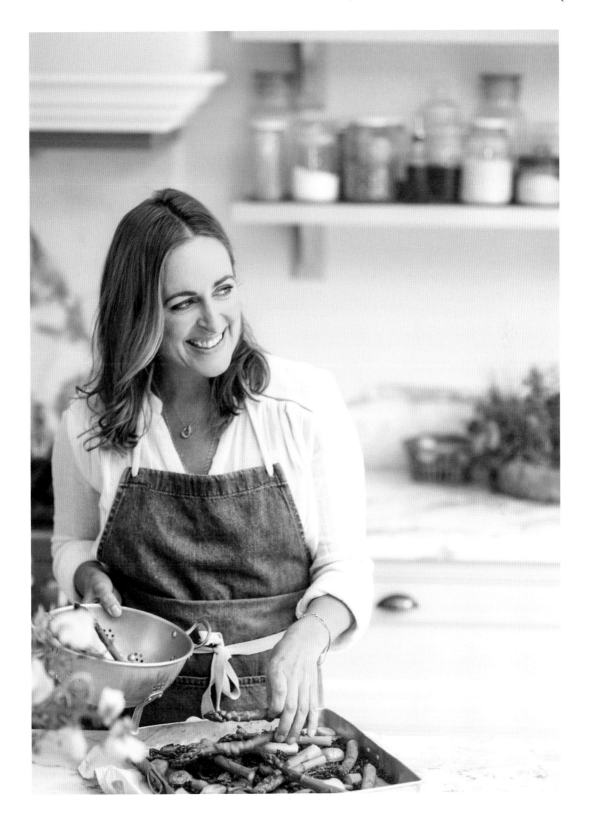

one-tray roasted spring salad
(vegan)

{Serves 2}

Just like the previous two roasted salads, I hope you'll agree that this is a winner of a dish. It will keep in the fridge for a lovely cold lunch the next day with some crumbled feta or goat's cheese.

200g new potatoes, halved

2 medium carrots, peeled, sliced lengthways, then cut into chunks

1 handful of tenderstem broccoli (approx. 100g)

1 bunch of asparagus (approx. 200g), woody ends removed

125g pre-cooked Puy lentils

1 handful of baby leaf spinach

sea salt and freshly ground black pepper

For the dressing

2 tablespoons extra virgin olive oil, plus extra for drizzling

2 tablespoons lemon juice, plus extra for serving

1 teaspoon Dijon mustard

a pinch of salt

Preheat the oven to 200°C /180°C fan.

Whisk together all the dressing ingredients until emulsified and smooth.

Tumble the potatoes and carrots on to a large roasting tray and drizzle over half the dressing. Turn a few times to coat the vegetables in the dressing, then roast for 25 minutes, until the potatoes are starting to brown and soften.

Add the broccoli, asparagus, lentils and the rest of the dressing. Mix or shake everything together again, then roast for a further 10 minutes.

When cooked, remove from the oven and tip the roasted salad into a serving bowl. Stir through the baby leaf spinach. The heat of the roasted vegetables and lentils will wilt it slightly.

Season with salt and pepper, then divide between bowls and drizzle over a little extra virgin olive oil and an additional squeeze of lemon.

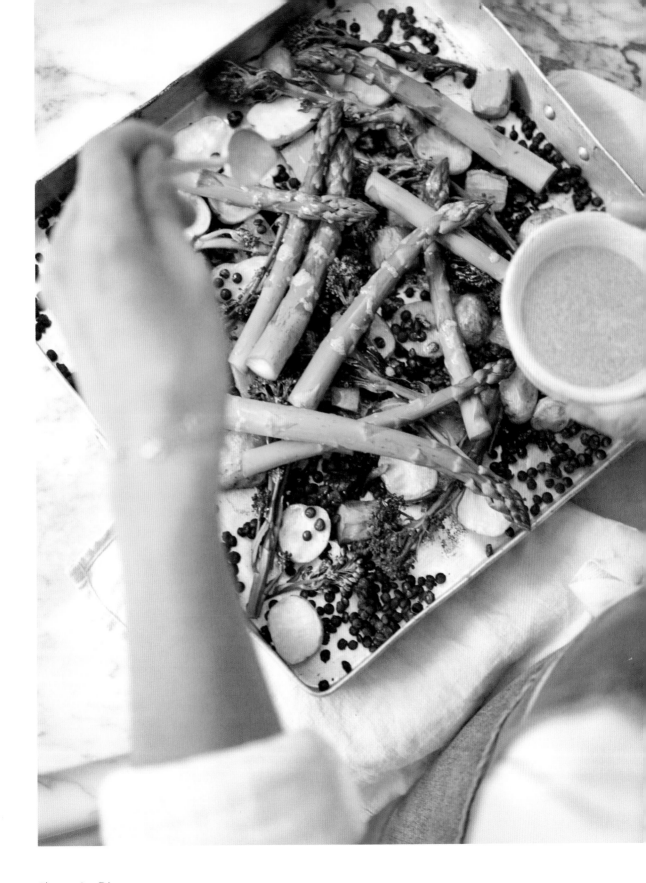

cauliflower & chickpea traybake with rocket & pickled red onion
(vegan)

This hearty plant-based dish is both a complete meal and a flavour sensation. The recipe will give you some extra dressing that will keep in the fridge for up to a week. I love it dolloped on to vegetables, salad, fish or chicken. It elevates most meals!

{Serves 2}

½ a cauliflower, cut into florets

2 tablespoons olive oil

1 teaspoon za'atar*

1 teaspoon sea salt

1 x 400g tin of chickpeas, drained and rinsed

½ teaspoon paprika

2 large handfuls of rocket

2 tablespoons toasted pine nuts

For the pickled red onion

¼ of a red onion, very finely sliced

2 tablespoons apple cider vinegar

1 teaspoon honey

freshly ground black pepper

For the dressing

75g tahini

4 tablespoons extra virgin olive oil

2 teaspoons apple cider vinegar

2 tablespoons water

1 teaspoon Dijon mustard

2 teaspoons honey

½ teaspoon sea salt

Preheat the oven to 220°C/200°C fan.

To make the pickled red onion, mix the red onion slices in a bowl with the vinegar, honey and a good grind of black pepper. Leave to marinate for at least 20 minutes, stirring every so often.

Put the cauliflower florets on to a large baking tray with 1 tablespoon of olive oil, the za'atar and ½ a teaspoon of salt. Roast in the oven for 20 minutes. After 5 to 10 minutes, remove the tray from the oven and use a spatula to gather the cauliflower to one side. Tip the chickpeas on to the other side and drizzle with another tablespoon of olive oil, the paprika and another ½ teaspoon of salt. Place back in the oven for the remaining 10 to 15 minutes.

Meanwhile, make the tahini dressing. Place all the ingredients in a bowl and whisk to combine.

Once the cauliflower and chickpeas are cooked, toss in a bowl with the rocket, drizzle with the dressing and add the pine nuts and drained pickled onions.

*
tip: If you don't like za'atar, use some ground cumin and coriander.

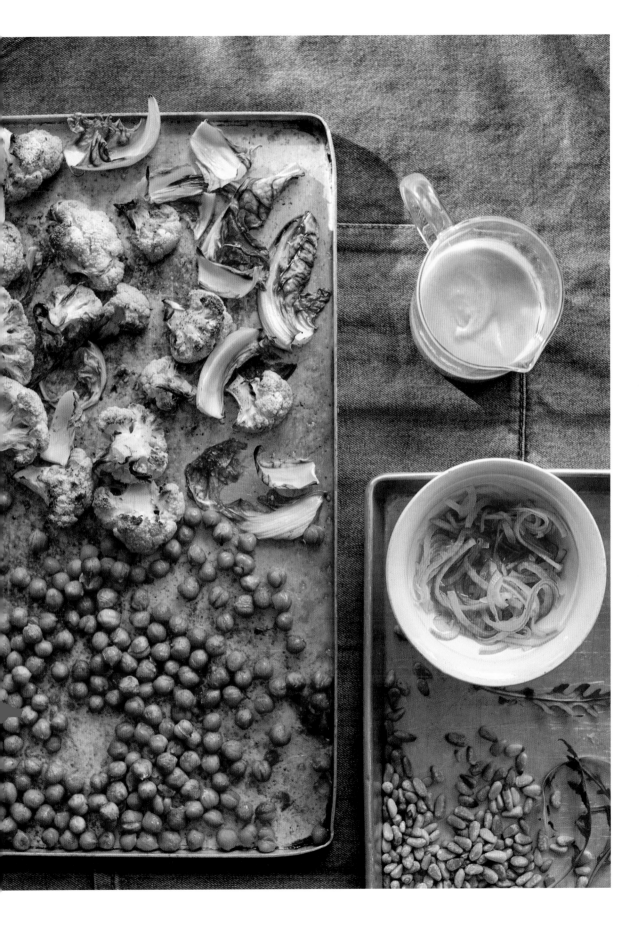

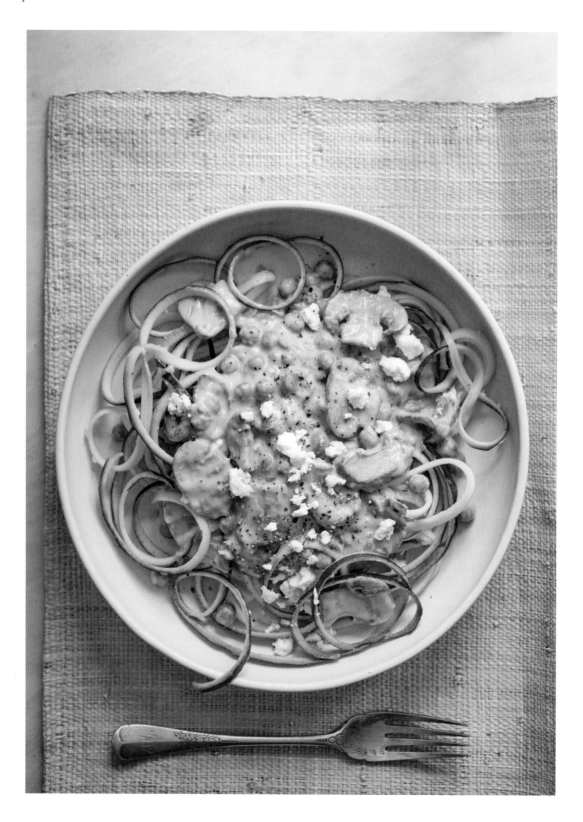

creamy
mushroom
pasta sauce

{Serves 4}

Is there anything more comforting than a bowl of creamy, garlicky pasta? This recipe evolved out of a little random experimentation one day. I didn't really expect it to work but it has become a staple recipe. If you can find wild mushrooms, that would elevate this into a very special dish.

1 red onion, peeled and thinly sliced

1 clove of garlic, peeled and crushed

olive oil

1 x 250g punnet of chestnut mushrooms, cleaned and sliced

1 x 400g tin of cannellini beans, drained and rinsed

100ml vegetable stock

75g feta

150g cooked peas

½ teaspoon Dijon mustard (optional)

sea salt and freshly ground black pepper

400g dried pasta of your choice, or courgetti

Lightly sauté the onions and garlic in a little olive oil for about 10 minutes, until soft. Add the mushrooms and continue cooking over a medium heat for 5 minutes, until golden.

Meanwhile, blend the cannellini beans with the vegetable stock and feta for 1 to 2 minutes in a high-speed blender. When smooth and creamy, pour over the mushrooms and onions, then add the peas and warm through. Stir in the mustard, if using, and season with salt and pepper to taste.

Meanwhile, cook your pasta or courgetti. Add the mushroom sauce, mix well, and serve.

tip: If you're plant-based, you can omit the feta (although you will also need to reduce the vegetable stock to avoid it all being too runny).

red pepper pasta sauce

(vegan)

{Serves 2}

I tend to choose legume pastas now they are more readily available – such as chickpea, or red lentil. They taste delicious, and have more protein than standard grain pastas, making them a complete and nutritionally balanced choice with very little extra effort. However, this sauce works well with whichever pasta you (or your family) particularly enjoy. Should you have any sauce left over, it can be stored in a jar in the fridge for 3 to 4 days, or frozen for a later date.

80g cashews (soaked for 2 hours in plenty of hot water, then drained)

2 roasted red peppers (from a jar or home-roasted, skins on)

2 sun-dried tomatoes

juice of ½ a lemon

3 tablespoons olive oil

1 teaspoon sea salt

a good grind of black pepper

To serve

200g pasta of your choice

fresh basil and Parmesan cheese (optional)

Blend all the ingredients together in a high-speed blender until smooth and creamy. You may need to add a dash of water if the sauce needs to be loosened a little.

Cook your pasta according to the packet instructions, and drain. Warm the sauce through in a saucepan, then stir it through the pasta.

Top with some torn fresh basil, if using, and some grated Parmesan or vegan alternative.

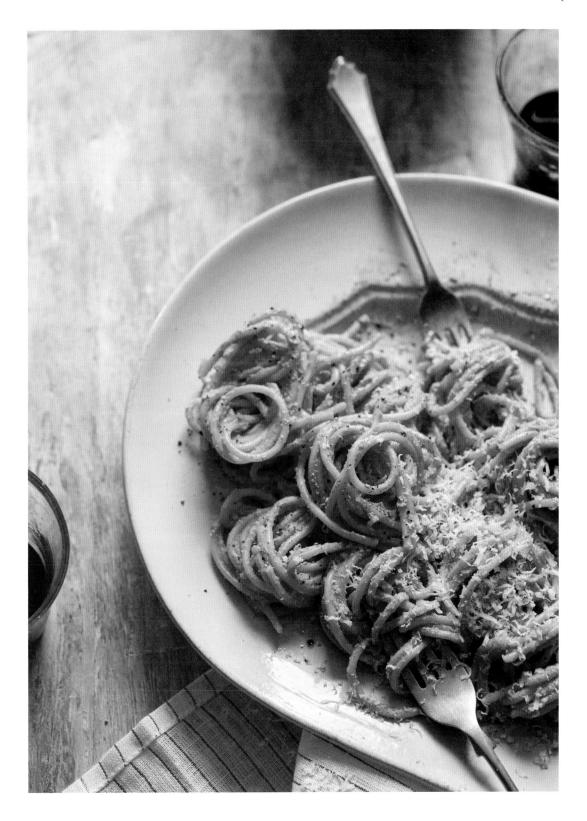

Chapter 3 ~ Dinner

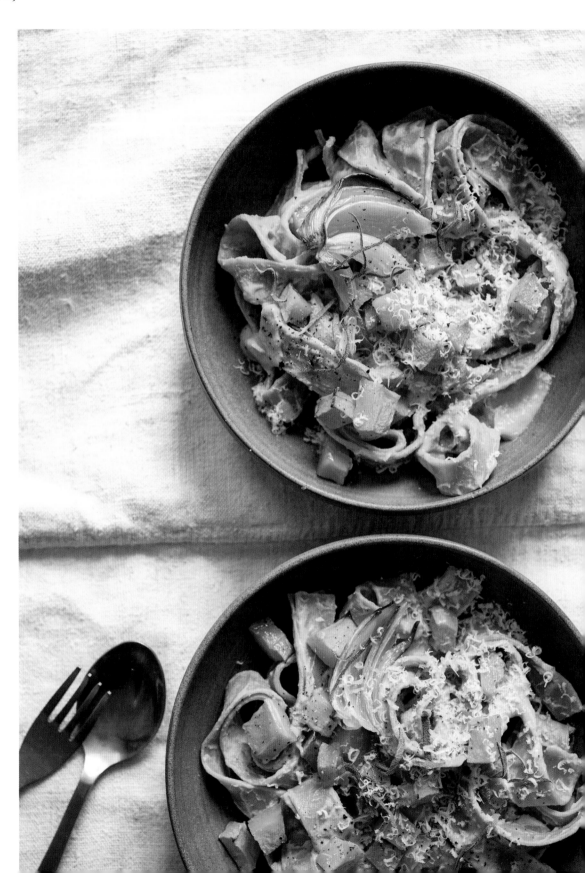

butternut, cashew & sage pasta sauce

(vegan)

{Serves 4}

Cashews, once soaked, blend really well into sauces to add creaminess (as well as healthy fats, protein and various essential minerals) and so are a useful ingredient if you are wishing to be more plant based or avoid dairy. Here I've blended them with roasted butternut squash and caramelized onions. This remains one of Willow's favourite sauces and I use it in many recipes. It's a winning recipe to have up your sleeve and a few portions stored in the freezer for busy days.

60g cashews

400ml hot water

1 medium butternut squash, peeled, deseeded and cut into bite-size pieces

1 onion, peeled and cut into wedges

sea salt and freshly ground black pepper

2 tablespoons olive oil

5 fresh sage leaves or 1 teaspoon dried sage (plus extra to garnish)

400g pasta of choice

a grating of Pecorino Romano or Parmesan (optional)

Preheat the oven to 220°C/200°C fan.

Pour the hot water over the cashews and leave to soak for 20 minutes.

Prepare your butternut squash and place in a roasting tray along with the onion wedges and a little salt and pepper. Drizzle with olive oil. Roast for 25 to 30 minutes, or until soft.

When cooked, allow to cool slightly, then take a third of the roasted vegetable mixture and blend in a high-speed blender with the sage leaves and the cashew/water mixture. Add a little more water if it is looking too thick to blend. You are aiming for a sauce consistency. Transfer to a pan and warm through gently.

Meanwhile, cook your pasta according to the packet instructions and drain. Stir the sauce into your cooked pasta of choice and add the rest of the vegetables and a sprinkling of fresh sage leaves. Top with grated Parmesan or Pecorino or vegan alternative (optional).

pad thai with
turmeric tofu
(vegan)

A filling and hearty vegan meal, perfect for sharing with friends. It's easy to switch around the vegetables, according to what you have available.

{Serves 4}

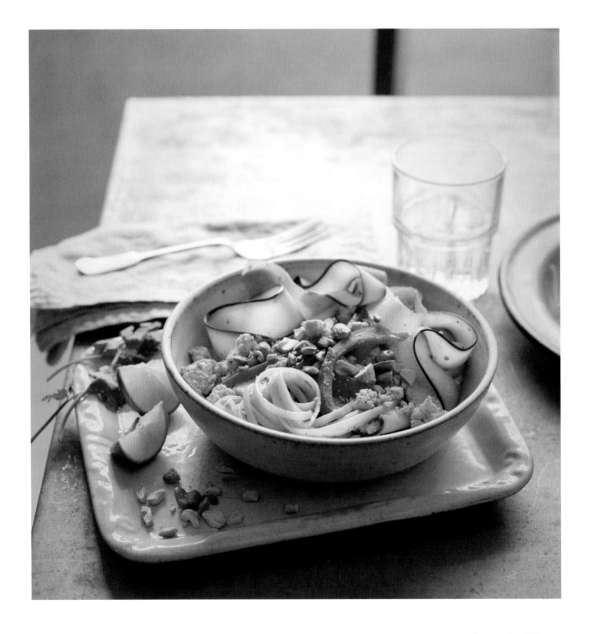

300g firm tofu

1½ teaspoons ground turmeric

sea salt and freshly ground black pepper

100g rice noodles

olive oil

1 clove of garlic, peeled and finely chopped

1 red chilli, finely diced

2 spring onions, sliced lengthways

1 red pepper, deseeded and cut into strips

1 pack of baby corn cobs, sliced lengthways

50g green beans, topped and tailed

1 small carrot, spiralized (or peeled into ribbons)

½ a courgette, spiralized (or peeled into ribbons)

For the sauce

2 tablespoons tamari

1 tablespoon rice vinegar

1 tablespoon maple syrup

2 teaspoons toasted sesame oil

1 tablespoon roasted almond/cashew or peanut butter

To top

a small handful of fresh coriander, roughly chopped

fresh lime juice

45g roasted cashews or peanuts, chopped

Use your hands to crumble the block of tofu into a small bowl. Add the turmeric and a good grind of black pepper. Stir well, then set aside.

Make the sauce by whisking all the ingredients together in a large bowl.

Next, prepare the noodles. Bring a medium pot filled with water to the boil, and cook the noodles according to the packet instructions. Drain and rinse, then toss the noodles through the dressing so they are well covered and have a chance to absorb some of the flavours.

Put a good glug of olive oil into a large saucepan or wok. Add the crumbled tofu to the pan and cook over a medium heat for 5 minutes or so. Sprinkle over a pinch of salt, then remove from the pan and set aside.

Using the same pan, add an additional couple of tablespoons of olive oil, along with the garlic, chilli and spring onions. Sauté over a medium heat for a couple of minutes. Add the red pepper, corn, green beans and carrots and sauté until tender, about 3 to 5 minutes, then add the courgettes and cook for a further 3 to 5 minutes.

Finally, add the noodles and the cooked tofu and stir through the vegetable mix to reheat.

Once hot, divide between bowls. Top with fresh coriander, squeeze over some lime juice and add the chopped peanuts or cashews.

SWEET
THINGS
4}

almond
scones
(gf)

Simple pleasures at their best. The joyful charm of a scone and jam. Best consumed straight from the oven, or freeze on the day they are made.

{Makes 12 small scones}

100g ground almonds

200g gluten-free plain flour

120ml milk (of your choice), plus a little extra for brushing over the top

1 large egg

2 teaspoons baking powder

3 tablespoons honey

1 tablespoon light olive oil (don't use extra virgin – you don't want to taste the olive oil)

200g raspberries or strawberries, mashed to a pulp with the back of a fork*

200g coconut yoghurt

almond butter (optional)

Preheat the oven to 200°C/180°C fan and line a baking tray with baking parchment.

Mix together the ground almonds, flour, milk, egg, baking powder, 2 tablespoons of honey and the olive oil in a large bowl to make a sticky dough.

Using damp hands, roll out 12 rough balls. Press the tops down slightly to flatten, and place on the baking tray. Brush with milk, and bake for 10 to 12 minutes, or until golden brown and slightly risen.

Mix the mashed berries with the remaining tablespoon of honey.

Allow the scones to cool slightly, then slice in half and top with a dollop of the berry mixture and some coconut yoghurt (or a little almond butter, if you like).

*
tip: Or use the berry chia jam recipe on page 56.

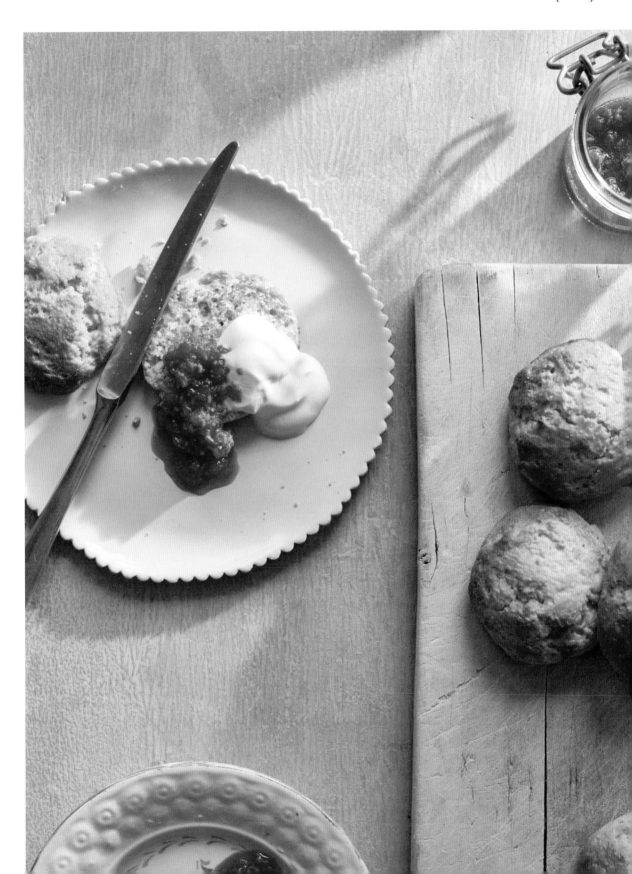

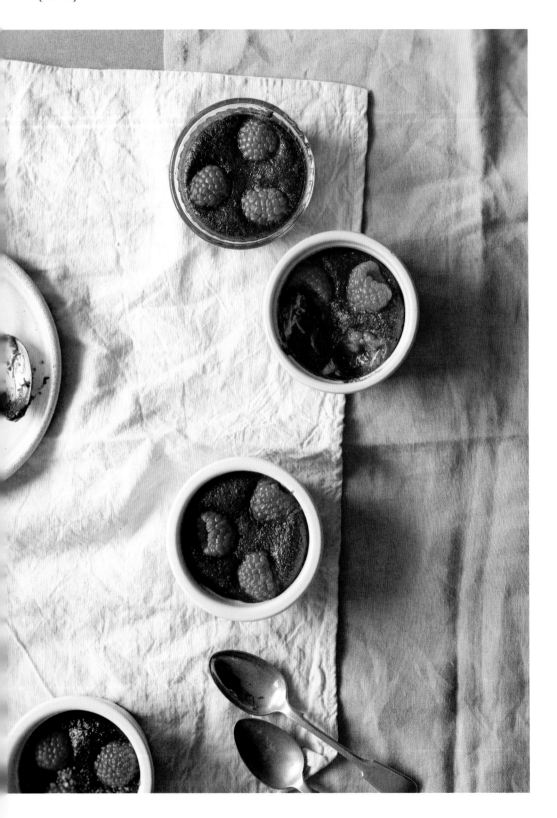

chocolate raspberry pots

{Makes 4}

Usually pudding in my house is a simple portion of fresh, seasonal fruit. However, sometimes the occasion calls for an extra course. And this rich, chocolate pot is where I would turn.

100g raspberries
(fresh ideally, but frozen
would also work)

3 large eggs, separated

100g organic dark
chocolate (85%), melted
and allowed to cool slightly

3 tablespoons honey

a pinch of sea salt

2 teaspoons vanilla extract

50g ground almonds

coconut yoghurt and
extra raspberries,
to serve (optional)

Preheat your oven to 180°C/160°C fan.

Divide the raspberries between four ramekins and place them in a roasting tray.

Whisk the egg yolks with the cooled, melted chocolate, honey, salt, vanilla extract and ground almonds. In a separate bowl, whisk the egg whites until they reach stiff peaks.

Fold small amounts at a time of the whisked egg whites into the chocolate mix, until well combined. Divide the mixture between the ramekins.

Carefully pour boiling water around the ramekins, creating a 'bain-marie'. You are aiming for the water to reach about three-quarters of the way up the sides of the ramekins.

Bake for 12 minutes. Be careful not to overbake – you want the centre to be very moist still.

Serve hot or cold, perhaps with a dollop of coconut yoghurt and a few extra raspberries.

honey roasted peaches & nectarines

{Serves 4}

The easiest summer pudding that there could possibly be. Roasting turns peaches and nectarines into an even more delicious feast (and works brilliantly even if the fruit are still a little under-ripe). I keep leftovers to enjoy the next morning for breakfast.

4 peaches

4 nectarines

3 teaspoons honey or maple syrup

1½ teaspoons vanilla extract

fresh raspberries and coconut yoghurt, to serve (optional)

Heat the oven to 200°C/180°C fan.

Halve the peaches and nectarines, and remove their stones. Place them, cut side up, on a baking tray. Whisk together the honey and vanilla extract, and drizzle over the cut fruit.

Bake for 20 to 30 minutes (a little longer if they are less ripe), or until soft and lightly caramelized.

Serve with fresh raspberries and a dash of coconut yoghurt, or simply as they are.

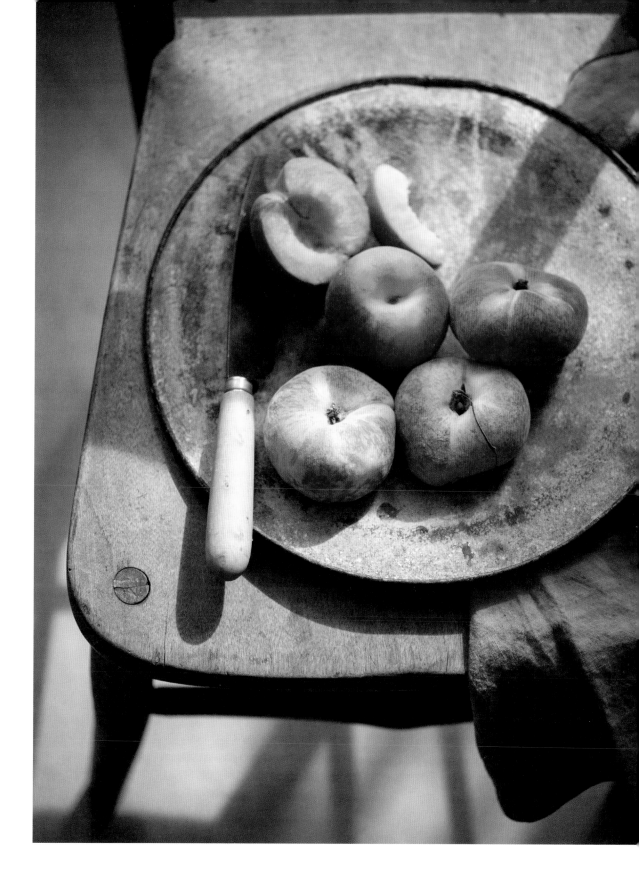

Chapter 4 ~ Sweet things

coconut
& almond
pear
crumble
(gf, vegan)

{Serves 4}

You can use any fruit to make a crumble, so opt for what is available and in season. Whilst this crumble topping differs from a traditional version, it is still a lovely option for a hassle free, mid-week pudding (or breakfast).

4 large, very ripe pears, washed, cored and diced (it's fine to leave the skins on)

2 teaspoons ground cinnamon

125g ground almonds

125g desiccated coconut

4 tablespoons maple syrup (or runny honey)

4 tablespoons light olive oil (avoid using your best extra virgin olive oil, it tastes too strong)

Preheat the oven to 200°C/180°C fan.

Throw the diced pears into an ovenproof dish, sprinkle with 1 teaspoon of cinnamon and mix together.

Mix together the ground almonds, coconut, maple syrup and olive oil in a bowl with the remaining teaspoon of cinnamon. It should have the consistency of damp sand.

Top the pears with the crumble mixture – no need to firm or pat it down. Bake for 25 to 30 minutes, or until golden brown.

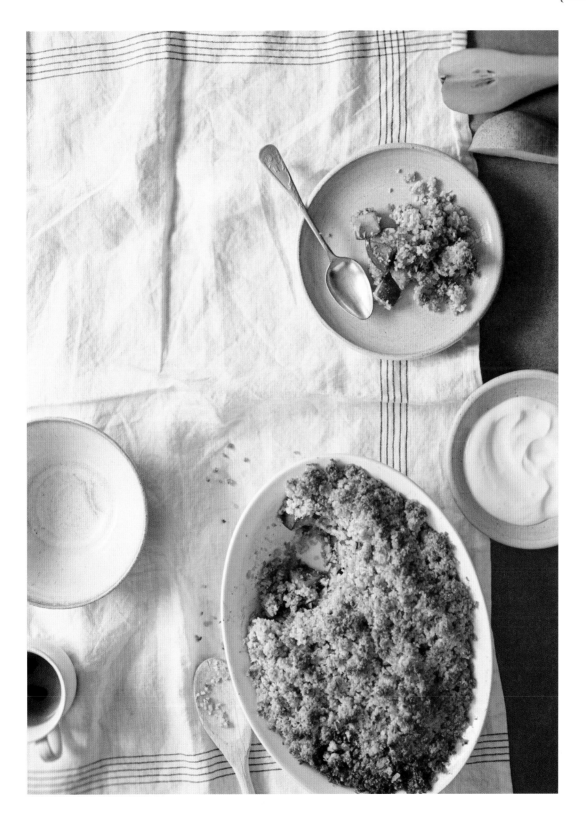

Chapter 4 ~ Sweet things

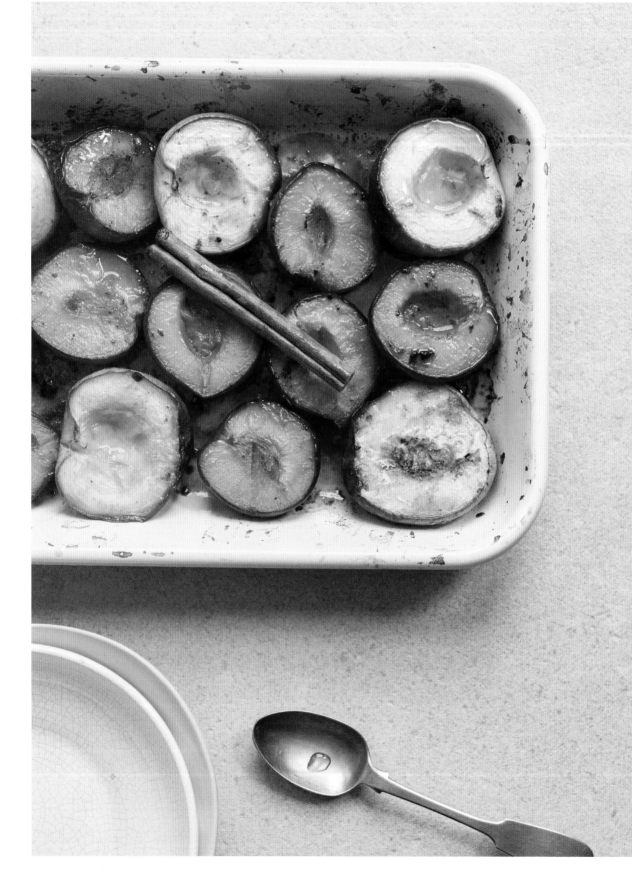

citrus spiced roasted plums

(vegan)

{Serves 4}

We have a very healthy plum tree that provides us with an enormous crop in the middle of summer. I make this with the ones that are just turning and need to be eaten. As simple as it sounds, it always feels and tastes decadent to me.

8 plums, (approx. 400g) halved and destoned

zest and juice of 1 large orange

¼ **teaspoon ground cinnamon**

1 teaspoon light olive oil (don't use extra virgin – you don't want to taste the olive oil)

Heat the oven to 200°C/180°C fan.

Toss all the ingredients together in a small ovenproof dish, so that the plums are well coated, then spread them out in a single layer.

Roast for 30 to 35 minutes, or until the plums are soft and gently burnished.

ginger & cacao squares

Reduce the amount of ginger if you don't like the strong flavour or if serving to little ones who might not be used to the spiciness. My colleague Rozzie introduced me to this recipe and it is such a good one, I make them all the time. Cacao powder is a little less processed than cocoa powder, but either works well for this recipe so use what you have.

{Makes 25 small squares}

150g pitted dates

100g oats

100g unsalted cashew nuts

4 tablespoons cacao or cocoa powder

80ml cold water

100g crystallized ginger

50g dark chocolate, melted (optional)

Blend the dates, oats, cashews and cacao powder in a food processor until they resemble breadcrumbs. Using the 'pulse' mode of the food processor, add the water bit by bit until the mixture starts to come together in clumps. You may need a little less than 80ml, you may need a little more.

Finally, add the crystallized ginger and pulse a couple more times to mix it through.

Tip the mixture into a baking dish or a 15cm square cake tin lined with baking parchment. Drizzle the top with a little melted dark chocolate, if you like.

Leave in the fridge for a few hours to set, then cut into bite-size squares.

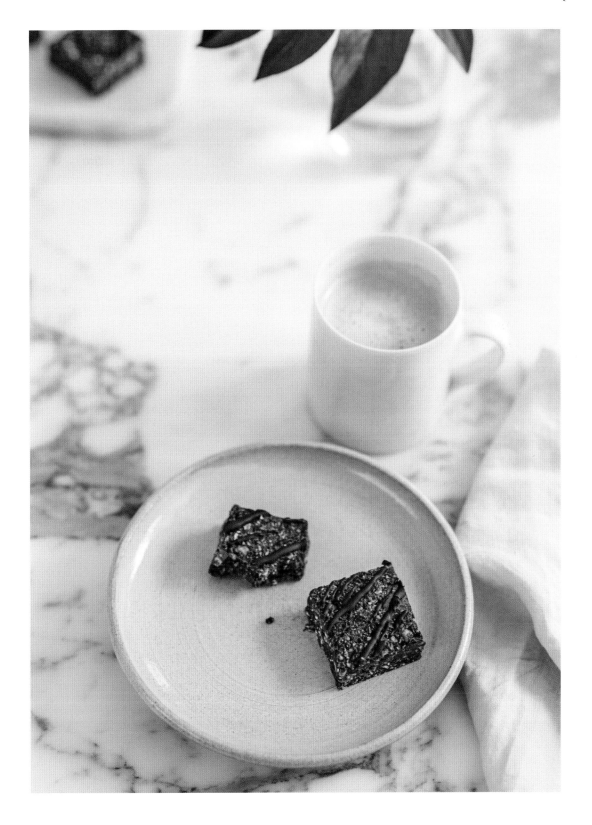

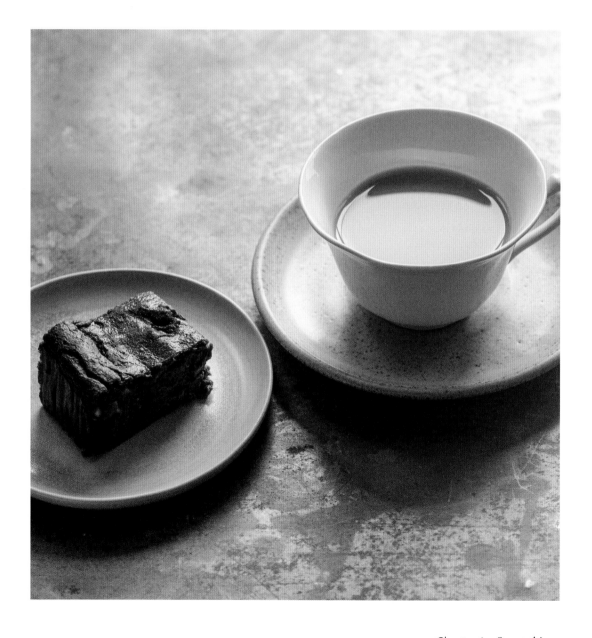

gooey courgette brownies

{Makes 12}

I grow courgettes each year, and usually end up with a large glut mid summer, so I am always thrilled to have the excuse to use them up for this recipe. Tahini and chocolate are an unexpected but complementary combination.

light olive oil, for greasing

150g pitted dates

2 medium courgettes, topped and tailed, then cut roughly into chunks

½ teaspoon sea salt

2 large eggs

60g tahini

3 heaped tablespoons cacao or cocoa powder

100g self-raising flour (I use Doves Farm Gluten Free)

Preheat the oven to 180°C/160°C fan. Grease and line an 18cm square baking tin.

Blend the pitted dates, courgettes, salt, eggs, tahini and cacao powder in a food processor until smooth. Tip into a mixing bowl, and fold in the flour.

Pour the brownie mix into the prepared tin and level the top. Bake for 25 to 30 minutes, or until the top and sides are dry. The middle should still be gooey.

Allow to cool completely, then slice into portions and remove from the tin. Due to the number of fresh ingredients in these brownies, they do need to be stored in the fridge (if they last that long!).

Optional
If you want to vary this base recipe, you could fold in any of the following:

~ 80g chopped walnuts, almonds, pistachios or hazelnuts

~ 80g chopped dark chocolate/chocolate chips

~ 80g dried cranberries or chopped dried apricots

~ 2 tablespoons maple syrup, if you prefer a sweeter version

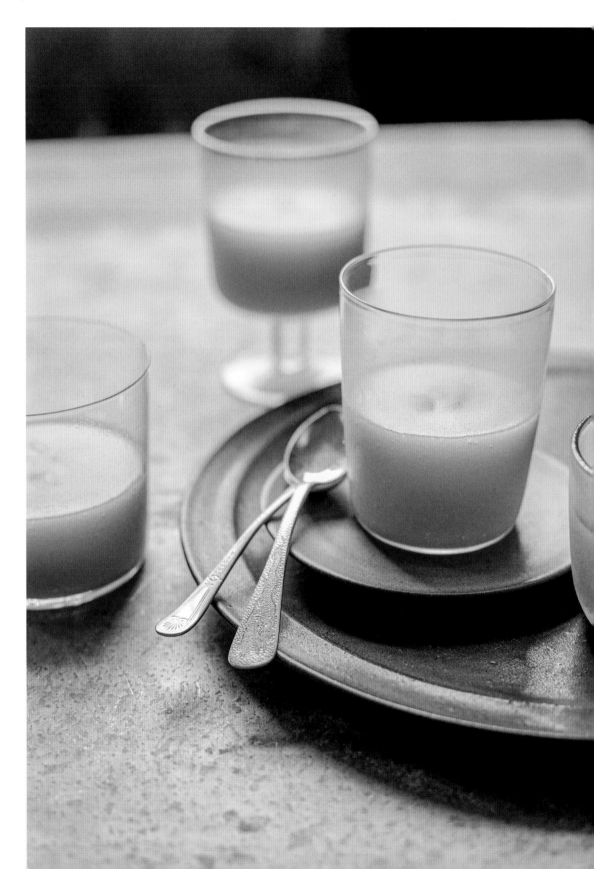

mango jelly

The great thing about mango is that it doesn't need any additional sweetness. I think this recipe, with just three ingredients, came about because I had frozen mango in the freezer and I was thinking of a sorbet but it morphed into jelly. And it works. Willow loves it. To make this recipe vegan, replace the gelatine with agar agar or Vege-Gel and follow the instructions for using these as they do differ.

{Serves 4}
(makes 4 x 150ml jellies)

500g mango flesh
(buying frozen mango makes this very easy)

100ml water

4 leaves gelatine*
(see notes below for vegan alternatives)

If the mango is frozen, allow it to thaw completely before using.

Blend the mango well until it becomes a thick, golden purée. Pass the resulting mixture through a sieve, using the back of a ladle or a flexible rubber spatula to press it down if necessary. This removes the fibrous strands of mango, which can interfere with the classical smooth texture of jelly, but you could skip this step if this doesn't bother you!

Measure the water into a small saucepan. Snip the gelatine leaves into small pieces and soak in the water for 15 minutes, until softened. Heat the water very gently, stirring continuously until the gelatine has dissolved. Stir the dissolved gelatine into the mango purée.

Spoon the mixture into a decorative bowl, or into four small glasses, and allow to set in the fridge.

*
tip: Vege-Gel and VegeSet – Measure 100ml of water into a small saucepan. Sprinkle over 2 teaspoons (1 sachet) of Vege-Gel or VegeSet and heat very slowly, stirring until it has dissolved. Stir into the mango purée as above.

peanut butter cookies

{Makes 10 to 12}

I have a bit of a thing for biscuits and so tend to avoid buying them otherwise I'd easily eat a whole packet in one go. But going to the effort of making these (admittedly they don't really require much effort) does slow me down as I want to savour them. I use coconut sugar as I love the flavour and it has slightly heathier properties than refined white sugar, but use whatever sugar you wish. I make these when I have lots of mouths to feed and there are never any left over.

250g peanut butter (I use chunky)*

150g sugar of choice (I use coconut)

1 large egg, lightly beaten

¼ teaspoon vanilla powder

2 tablespoons chocolate chips (optional)

Preheat the oven to 200°C/180°C fan. Line two baking sheets with baking parchment.

Put all the ingredients into a bowl and stir well to combine.

Spoon tablespoons of the mixture on to the lined baking sheets, leaving space for the cookies to spread. Bake in the oven for 8 to 10 minutes.

Leave to cool on the trays, then move to a rack to cool completely. They will keep in an airtight tin for up to 3 days.

*
tip: When buying peanut (or any nut) butter, I always opt for ones that don't include palm oil and have the fewest ingredients.

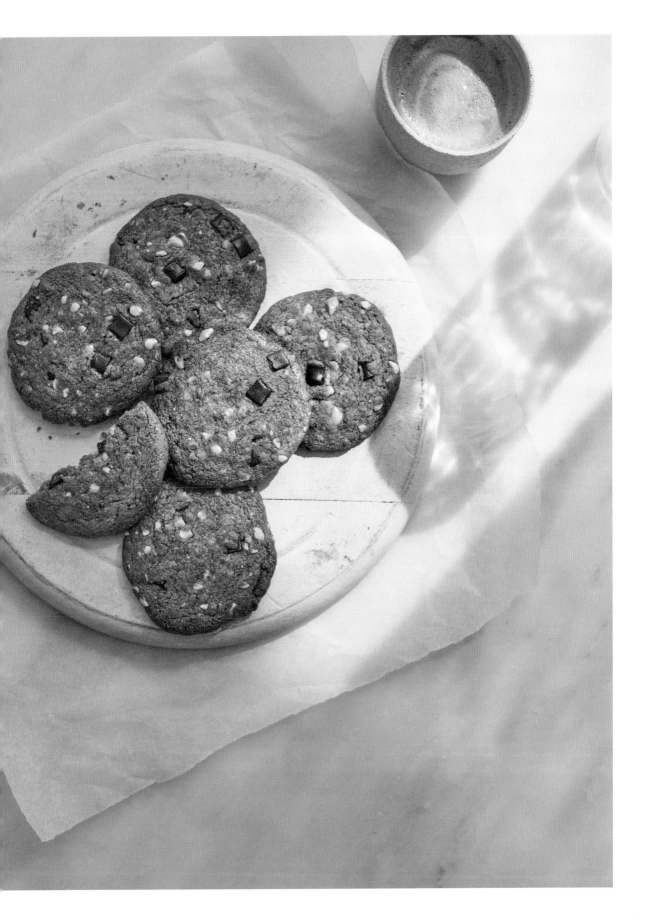

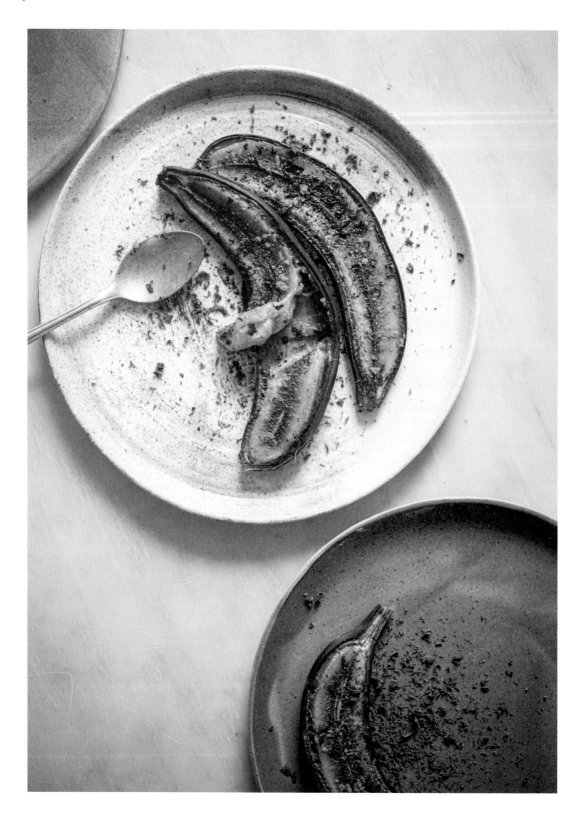

baked bananas with chocolate cinnamon

{Serves 2}

I confess to being rather lazy when it comes to puddings or desserts. It's the part of the meal where I have run out of enthusiasm and effort and I'm usually full anyway. Hence I don't have them often. However, I know that many people still enjoy puddings and so I'll make them but they have to be incredibly simple. I remember when I first tasted baked bananas. It was on holiday and a friend's parents wrapped them in foil and cooked them on the BBQ. This is my quicker and easier version but no less sublime.

2 **bananas** (not overly ripe)

½ **teaspoon ground cinnamon**

1 **square of dark chocolate**

Preheat the oven to 200°C/180°C fan and line a baking tray with baking parchment.

Slice the bananas in half lengthways – keeping the skin on – and place them on the tray skin side down. Sprinkle with the cinnamon and bake for 10 to 15 minutes, or until cooked to your liking.

Once out of the oven, grate over the dark chocolate and serve.

roasted fruit salad

We so often roast trays of vegetables, but why not fruit? I've done it many times now and it's truly wonderful! Far more flavourful than the raw ingredients. Give it a try.

{Serves 4}

4 plums, destoned and chopped into bite-size pieces

2 bananas, peeled and chopped

2 apples, cored and chopped

1 punnet of blueberries

1 tablespoon light olive oil (don't use extra virgin – you don't want to taste the olive oil)

1 tablespoon honey or maple syrup

½ teaspoon ground cinnamon

½ teaspoon ground ginger

Preheat the oven to 200°C/180°C fan. Line a large baking tray with baking parchment.

Mix all the ingredients together in a large bowl, then transfer to the prepared baking tray and roast for 20 to 25 minutes.

Equally delicious eaten hot or cold.

Note
This recipe works with a wide variety of fruit combinations, but is best with the following 'formula':

~ A stone fruit (plums/nectarines/peaches/cherries)
+
~ A hard fruit (apples/pears)
+
~ A berry (blueberries/raspberries/strawberries)
+
~ Bananas, which add a delicious, caramel sweetness when roasted

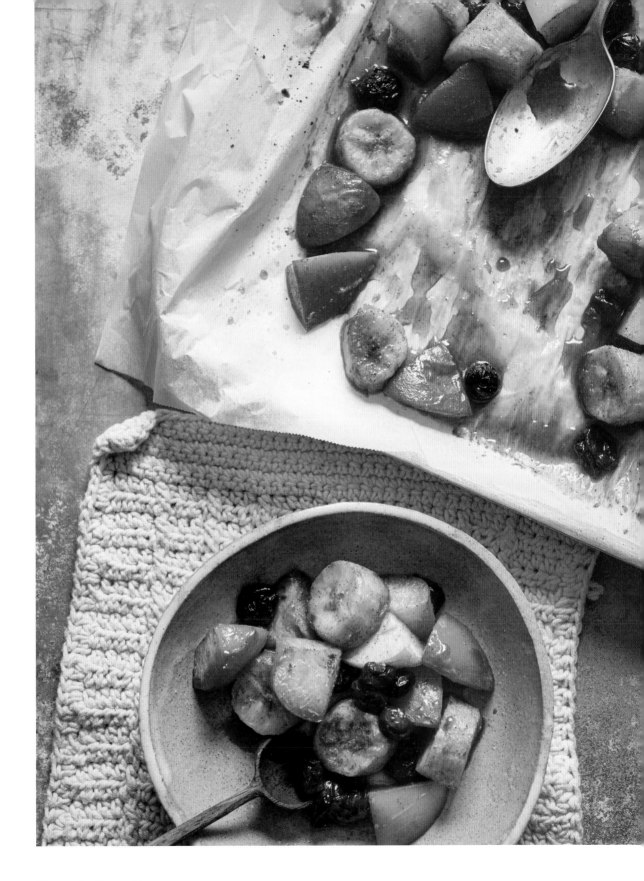

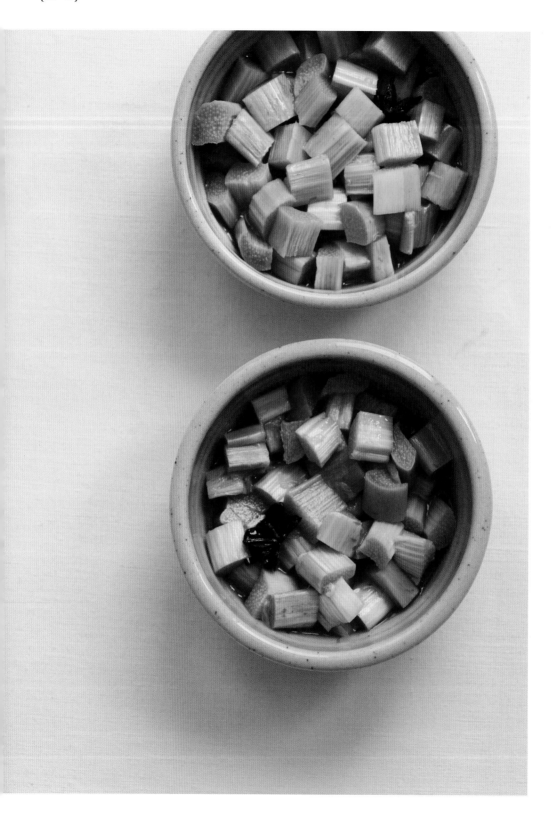

rhubarb & star anise crumble pot

(gf, vegan)

{Serves 2}

Rhubarb is the first vegetable to appear in our garden in March and for me, it's a celebration after the long, barren winter. It couldn't be easier to harvest, chop and stew and paired with star anise, makes a terrific pudding. I use a little fresh orange juice and a little coconut sugar to sweeten it. The topping is naturally gluten free (use gluten free oats if you are sensitive) and can of course be used with any stewed fruits. It's a light, not too sweet dessert (or breakfast as has occurred once or twice in our house).

250g rhubarb

juice of 1 orange
(around 50ml)

30g sugar of choice,
I use coconut

1 star anise, broken in half

Crumble topping

25g oats

25g almonds, whizzed into
small chunks (not too fine)

2 large pinches of ground
cinnamon

a large pinch of sea salt

1 teaspoon melted coconut
oil or light olive oil

1 tablespoon maple syrup
or honey

Preheat the oven to 200°C/180°C fan.

Wash the rhubarb, top and tail it, and cut the stems into cubes of equal size. In a large bowl, toss the rhubarb with the orange juice, coconut sugar, and star anise. Divide between two little ovenproof pots, making sure each has a star anise half, and roast for 10 minutes.

Meanwhile, using the same bowl, mix the oats, almond bits, cinnamon, salt, coconut or olive oil and maple syrup. Lay half the crumble mix on top of each cooked rhubarb pot.

Put back into the oven and cook for another 30 to 40 minutes, until the crumble looks crunchy and golden.

ice lollies

When I was little, I'd make ice lollies out of fruit-flavoured cordial. These days I use fresh fruit and opposite are two of my regular combinations, but please don't let my creations hold you back. Use whatever fruits you or your loved ones enjoy. They couldn't be easier and still count towards our five a day.

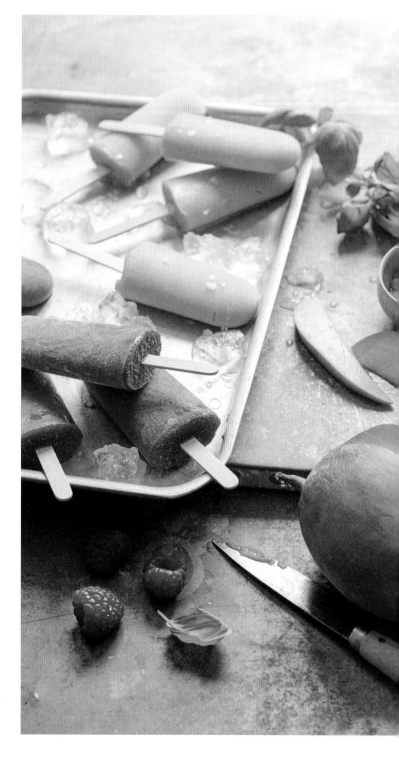

coconut and mango ice lollies

{Makes about 4 lollies}
(depending on the size
of your moulds)

1 medium mango (fresh or frozen – approx.
280g mango flesh)

½ teaspoon ground turmeric (optional)

a grind of black pepper

100g coconut yoghurt

1 tablespoon maple syrup (if needed)

Blitz the mango pieces, turmeric (if using)
and pepper in a food processor or equivalent,
until smooth.

Pour the mango into a jug and stir through the
coconut yoghurt. This is a good time to have
a little taste to see if the mixture needs some
maple syrup for added sweetness (to your
own personal taste) – if so, add it and stir
to incorporate.

Pour the mixture into lolly moulds, add
sticks if you are using them, and leave to
freeze overnight.

raspberry and yoghurt ice lollies

{Makes about 4 lollies}
(depending on the size
of your moulds)

300g raspberries

4 fresh basil or mint leaves (optional)

1–2 tablespoons maple syrup (if needed)

100g Greek yoghurt (or coconut yoghurt)

Blitz the raspberries with the basil or mint
leaves (if using). Taste to see if the mixture
needs a little sweetening, and if so, add
1–2 tablespoons of maple syrup.

Pour into a jug, add the yoghurt, and gently
stir to create a mottled/marbled mix.

Pour the mixture into lolly moulds, add sticks
if you are using them, and leave to freeze
overnight.

thanks

Writing a cookbook was a long-held dream for me. Having collected and devoured pages and pages of them since my early twenties, I was surprisingly clueless as to how much work and just how many people it took to create one. My fourth endeavour has been a lengthy process, and both challenging and immensely rewarding. Naturally it has been a huge team effort.

I am forever indebted to my publisher, Louise Moore at Michael Joseph, for giving me the opportunity to share my knowledge and passion and continue to help more people to eat well and feel better. It means a great deal to me to continue working with such an esteemed publishing house and talented people. Special thanks go to Fenella Bates, Sarah Fraser, Emma Plater, Nick Lowndes, Ione Walder, Beth O'Rafferty, Clare Parker and Gail Jones.

The photoshoot is a really fun and creative part of the process and this one was a particularly magical three weeks, with a truly supportive, collaborative, inspiring and hardworking team. Abundant thanks to Libby Silbermann and her assistants, Sophie Pryn, Saskia Sidey, Sophie Foot and Olivia Williamson, who calmly and brilliantly brought my book to life. Louie Waller, whose taste is exquisite, provided the dreamiest props. Susan Bell, who calmly orchestrated the shoot, and with her beautiful eye and warmth, made the book blossom. And Susan's lovely assistants, Maria Aversa, Kristina Sälgvik and Aloha Bonser-Shaw. Finally, thanks so much to Philippe Tholimet and Sjaniël Turrel for making this very tired mama feel pretty for a day.

Huge thanks to all of my followers on Instagram and Facebook for their kind words, photographs of my recipes, feedback and enthusiasm for my work.

And then there are the individuals who made it possible for this book to exist and enabled me to work while also being a mother. I am eternally grateful to my support system – my collaborator and friend Rozzie Yoxall, my creative director Candida Boddington, my associate Nicola Moore and assistant Clemmie Macpherson. Also, Stephanie Yates, Suzi Fryer, Mia Watts, Hazel Hurle, Mark Duffield and Andy Clarke. And all of my friends and family who have my back from afar, yet I don't get to spend enough time with.

Thanks to my rock, Nick Jenkins, who makes every day better.

This book is dedicated to my daughter, Willow, who has challenged every aspect of healthy eating, cooking and wellbeing while also liberating me and teaching me how wonderfully simple it can be. She is magnificent!

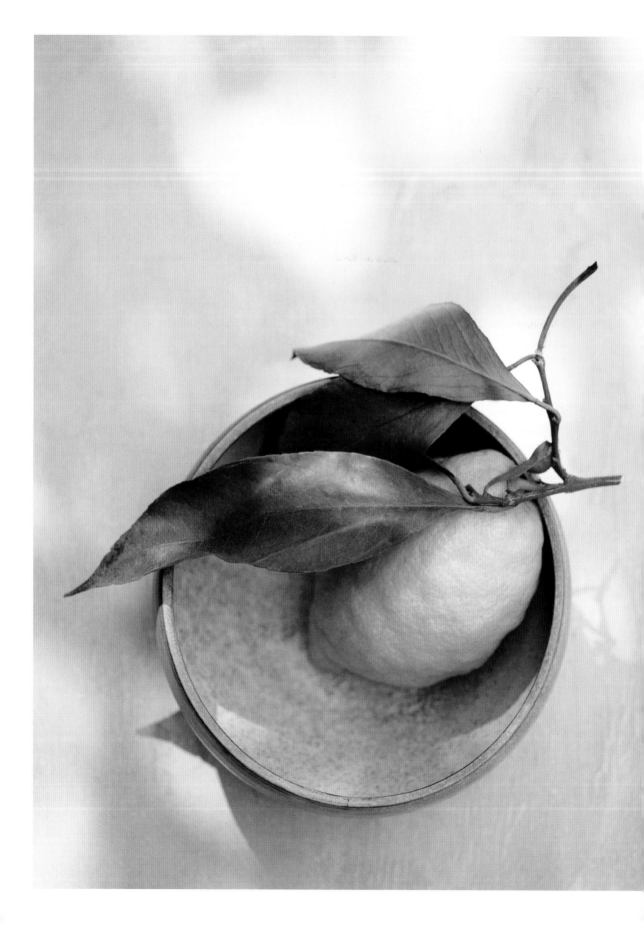

index

MICHAEL JOSEPH

UK | USA | Canada | Ireland | Australia
India | New Zealand | South Africa

Michael Joseph is part of the Penguin Random House group of companies
whose addresses can be found at global.penguinrandomhouse.com

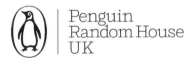

First published 2019
001

Text copyright © Amelia Freer, 2019
Photography copyright © Susan Bell, 2019

The moral right of the author has been asserted

Colour reproduction by Rhapsody Ltd
Printed and bound by Livonia Print, Latvia

A CIP catalogue record for this book is available from the British Library

ISBN: 978–0–241–41468–2

BY THE SAME AUTHOR: Eat. Nourish. Glow.

Cook. Nourish. Glow.

Nourish and Glow: The 10-Day Plan

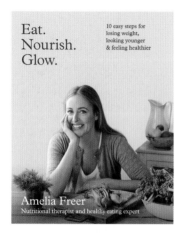
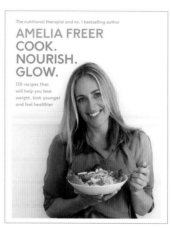
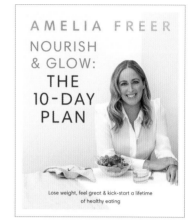

FIND ME AT: www.ameliafreer.com

Instagram: @ameliafreer

Facebook: Amelia Freer Nutrition

Email: info@ameliafreer.com

**WOMEN
SUPPORTING
WOMEN**

Changing Young Lives
Building Futures

10 per cent of Amelia's proceeds from this book will be donated to Women Supporting Women, an initiative from The Prince's Trust, to ensure that no young woman is left behind. Women Supporting Women is a passionate community who are committed to changing the lives of young women, giving more young women in the UK the skills and confidence to live, learn and earn. We provide the right help to nurture, empower and inspire young women to build their own positive futures through employment, self-employment, education or training. For more information please visit https://www.princes-trust.org.uk/support-our-work/major-gifts/women-supporting-women